CONTRACT 200?

A GP's GUIDE TO
EARNING THE MOST

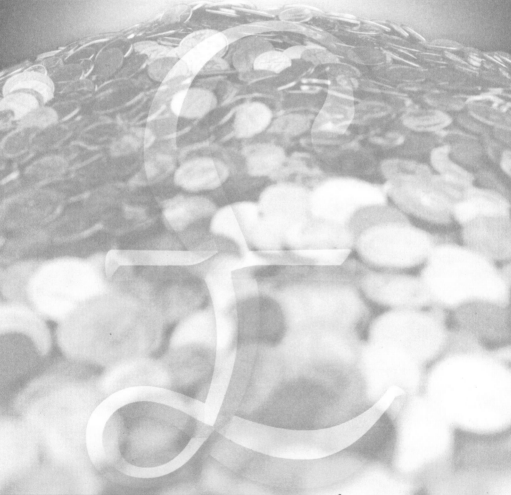

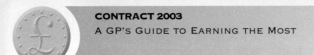

BUTTERWORTH HEINEMANN:

COMMISSIONING EDITOR: Heidi Allen

DEVELOPMENT EDITOR: Kim Benson

PROJECT MANAGER: Nina Keegan, Lucy Thorburn

DESIGN/PRODUCTION: Steve Green

CONTRACT 2003

A GP'S GUIDE TO EARNING THE MOST

SIMON CARTWRIGHT MB BS MRCGP DCH DRCOG
White Horse Medical Practice,
Faringdon, Oxfordshire

GLYNIS BUCKLE
Practice Manager
Albany House Medical Centre
Wellingborough
Northants

MICHAEL GILBERT
Financial Accountant
RMT
Newcastle-upon-Tyne

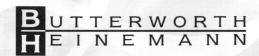
BUTTERWORTH
HEINEMANN

EDINBURGH LONDON NEW YORK OXFORD
PHILADELPHIA ST LOUIS SYDNEY TORONTO 2003

BUTTERWORTH HEINEMANN
An imprint of Elsevier Limited

© 2003 Elsevier Limited

'Advanced Access' is reproduced by kind permission of Sir John Oldham and the National Primary Care Development Team.

Published 2003

ISBN 0 7506 8796 7

British Library Cataloguing in Publication Data
A catalogue record for this book is available from the British Library.

Library of Congress Cataloging in Publication Data
A catalog record for this book is available from the Library of Congress.

Note
Medical knowledge is constantly changing. As new information becomes available, changes in treatment, procedures, equipment and the use of drugs become necessary. The author/contributors and the publishers have taken great care to ensure that the information given in this text is accurate and up to date. However, readers are strongly advised to confirm that the information, especially with regard to drug usage, complies with the latest legislation and standards of practice.

Printed in Spain (Graphycems)

The
Publisher's
policy is to use
**paper manufactured
from sustainable forests**

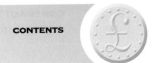

CONTENTS

PREFACE viii

INTRODUCTION 1

The history of the new contract for general practice 2
The financial potential 3

THE IDEAL PRACTICE 5

Ethos 5
Practice structure 7
Information Technology 10
Accountancy 14
Business Planning 17
Working practices 21
Diversity 22
Responsibility for income generation 26
Potential income 28

DIVERSITY 31

GMS – The range of services 31
Private work 35
Setting up a private service – the vasectomy clinic 43
Working with other practices 46
GP specialists 48
Summary – achieving a balance 49

SKILL MIX 51

Traditional models 51
Financial perspective 52
Changing practice workforce structures 54
Summary 59

PRACTICE SIZE 61

Introduction 61
Economy of scale 61
Other staff 62
Medical staff 62
Downside of the large practice 63
Practice versus partnership 63
Opportunities for change 64
Summary 65

OUT-OF-HOURS .... .67

    Introduction .... .67
    How to opt out .... .68
    Cost comparison with other income streams .... .69
    Working for the PCO doing out-of-hours .... .69
    Competition for GPs wanting to provide out-of-hours .... .70
    Bidding to provide out-of-hours .... .71
    Pricing out-of-hours .... .72
    Co-operatives as providers of out-of-hours after December 2004 .... .72
    Summary .... .73

QUALITY .... .75

    Introduction .... .75
    The key to success .... .76
    Method of payment .... .77
    Computer templates .... .79
    Exclusions (exception reporting) .... .79
    Ghost patients .... .80
    Multiple pathology .... .80
    Establishing a structured annual review .... .81
    Monitor your progress .... .82
    Individual clinical areas .... .82
    Organisational quality indicators .... .101
    Patient experience .... .105
    Additional services (additional payments for quality) .... .105
    Holistic care payments .... .106
    Quality practice payment .... .106
    Access .... .107
    Rising up the quality ladder .... .107
    Troubleshooting .... .108

ENHANCED SERVICES .... .109

    Introduction .... .109
    Finances .... .109
    Types of service .... .110
    Calculated profit versus actual profit: the differences ...... .114
    The workforce sponge: economies of scale .... .115
    Diversity .... .115
    The enhanced services: how much are they worth? .... .117

PERSONAL MEDICAL SERVICES (PMS) 123

    Sources of advice 125
    Making the proposal 125
    The financial benefits 126
    Switching back to GMS from PMS 127

ACCESS 129

    Introduction 129
    Definition of access 129
    Finances 129
    Meeting the targets for access (Sir John Oldham) 130
    Monitoring 138
    Troubleshooting 138

SENIORITY 141

APPENDIX 1: COMPUTER RESOURCES 143

    EMIS 143
    Torex 144
    InPractice Systems 144

APPENDIX 2: SAMPLE MEDICO-LEGAL REPORT 145

APPENDIX 3: VASECTOMY CLINIC PAPERWORK 151

APPENDIX 4: PATIENTS' SATISFACTION QUESTIONNAIRES .159

    GPAQ 160
    IPQ 164

INDEX 167

PREFACE

General practice has undergone the most radical change since the birth of the National Health Service in 1948. The new General Medical Services (GMS) contract has fundamentally altered the way GP practices work, not least in the way they are paid.

In these early days of the new contract there has been much speculation about how best to run things and to make a good living from being a doctor. Many GPs find this a confusing time, and others worry about falling incomes and uncertainty.

With the new GMS contract being in its infancy, it is timely to take a look at general practice finance, not only from the NHS perspective but from that other important area, private practice.

This book is concerned with those aspects of a GP's life that have an influence on profits: income and expenses, and the balancing act between workload and quality of life. GMS contract payments are dealt with for the first time, and non-GMS work and private work are also explored. Aimed primarily at GP principals in GMS practices, as well as their practice managers, there are also sections on Personal Medical Services (PMS). GPs considering moving into a GMS practice would also find this book useful.

The advice of a specialist medical accountant and a practice manager has been sought throughout. Their tips are interspersed among the chapters.

This guidebook will help you to steer your way through the maze of practice finance, towards maximising the bottom line – profit!

Simon Cartwright
June 2003

ACKNOWLEDGEMENTS

I have been very lucky in writing this book to have been offered much advice, freely given, from a rich diversity of sources. Special thanks are due to:

Mike Gilbert and Glynis Buckle, Robin Stride of Doctor magazine, Andreas Lambrianou of Pricare – for information on PMS, Heidi Allen & Kim Benson at Elsevier, Dr John Oldham of the National Primary Care Development Team – for the work on Advanced Access, Virginia Bushell, my practice manager, and the partners & staff of The White Horse Medical Practice, Faringdon, Oxfordshire.

INTRODUCTION

Running a General Medical Practice in Britain is like running a small business; there are staff to employ, invoices flying about, profit and loss to consider, premises to deal with. But while GPs are therefore businessmen and women, very few like to think of themselves as such.

GPs see themselves as inhabiting the gentler world of the healing arts. There is no requirement for a business studies qualification to enter medical school. Nor is there any focus on finance and accounting in the undergraduate medical curriculum. And in medical practice in general, there is little sign of the ethos of financial wealth generation, unlike that in, say, the legal world.

In fact, many GPs are a little embarrassed, ashamed even, to think about how they might maximise their income. When other health care workers earn so little and the bulk of GPs' income comes from the taxpayer, it is hardly surprising. I earn quite enough already, they say. I'll just get on with being a doctor.

But like many other groups of people, GPs are not unusual in wanting to earn a good living. It is not wrong to try and run the most efficient practice and to earn a high income. In fact, there is nothing evil in striving to be the highest-earning GP in Britain, as long as you do so within the law and without compromising the medical care of your patients.

So, if you want to cast off the sackcloth and ashes and take a look at how you can improve your income, this is the book for you!

Some practices have traditionally been high earning, while others have been exactly the opposite. What is it that makes these high-earners so successful?

Under the old GMS contract, GPs with high earnings tended to run large list sizes, to rigorously claim all fees and allowances, to have high outside earnings and to be first-movers into new, government-led initiatives often laced with inducement money. There are lessons in this pattern of behaviour for any GP wanting to join the list of top-earning practices. Although the new contract for general practice has opened up different opportunities for income generation, many of the old principles still apply. Throughout this book, these principles will be explored, with worked examples and practical hints on implementing them in your own practice.

Furthermore, the new contract has radically altered the way general medical services are paid for, leaving GPs to work out the best ways to make a living. This overhaul of fees is both threatening and exciting – at once a risk to time-honoured working patterns and, at the same time, a chance to adapt and prosper. This book explores the new contract with the aim of helping GPs to maximise profit. With the help of a specialist medical accountant and a practice manager fluent with practice finance, the following pages will show how practices can join that elite band of high-earners.

THE HISTORY OF THE NEW CONTRACT FOR GENERAL PRACTICE

The need for a new contract for general practice was first realised by the profession as long ago as 1990. Under the old GMS contract, there was too much emphasis placed on rewarding high-volume, low-quality medicine. Practices wanting to increase profits from GMS were obliged to try to attract more and more patients onto their lists, in order to boost capitation fees. The consequence of chasing the big list was that the pressure on appointments was directly proportional to the success in recruiting new patients. Older patients attracted a higher capitation fee but were harder work, as were those a long way from the surgery for whom rural mileage was paid.

Other bizarre examples of the old contract's inadequacy abound. A high turnover of patients boosted new registration fees but diminished continuity of care. Minor surgery fees were identical for both the 30-minute toenail removal and the 10-second cryotherapy of a wart. In fact, GPs could earn as much from a single session of wart freezing as they could from an entire year's worth of running a diabetes clinic, and nothing was paid for managing the secondary prevention of coronary heart disease!

Apart from leading to frustration and overwork, the consequence of the old contract's peculiarity was that earnings from GMS hit an effective ceiling. Partnerships were limited in their earnings by the amount of time available to the GPs for seeing patients, while GP numbers were capped by the Medical Practices Committee. Once surgeries reached saturation point, there was no incentive for working harder, and no chance of increasing earnings.

This frustration was picked up by the General Practitioners Committee of the British Medical Association. A vote by the profession in early 2001 resulted in a promise of mass resignation if a new contract was not negotiated between the BMA and the government. Talks resulted in a framework document being accepted, followed, after much last-minute haggling, by the new contract for GMS we have today. Implementation of the new contract will require primary legislation to pass through government and will not be complete until April 2004.

Most of the contract has, however, been implemented. GPs are now faced with the daunting task of working within the constraints of a new system of rewards, requirements and opportunities. Maintaining any business in a changing world is never easy, but the financial health of your practice will be easier to achieve with the help and advice in this book.

THE FINANCIAL POTENTIAL

Analyses of GPs' income under the old GMS contract showed that the average practice would generate profits per whole-time partner of between £40,000 and £90,000 a year. The wide range was attributable to many variables, but the upper limit was difficult to achieve, and only reached by a few.

The new GMS contract has placed the high income within the sights of many more practices. New opportunities for income generation have been created, and practices have effectively been given more control over how to manage profit and loss.

It is not unreasonable now to expect incomes per whole-time partner to reach £120,000. Certainly, figures such as these are achievable with a combination of the new GMS contract and existing private and dispensing incomes.

Aiming for the top earnings as a GP partner in a GMS practice requires organisational change. The money will not simply roll in to the practice bank account for just working hard as a good doctor. Nor will high income be achieved by continuing to grind away under the system that suited the old GMS contract. But if you are prepared for change, to embrace new opportunities and to set up the right systems, you can expect to be rewarded with those six-figure sums GPs only dreamed of under the Red Book.

The very highest incomes in general practice are achievable only by making financial wealth a high priority. Not all doctors want to do this; they put patient care and their own quality of life higher up the priority ladder. The extent to which a practice pursues high income is a decision for the partners, and will be reached after some considerable soul-searching.

In this book, the purpose of highlighting the financial possibilities of the new GMS contract is to show what can be achieved. The following pages explain in more detail how to attain high financial rewards under the different sections of the new contract. Some will seem easy, some possible and others difficult to achieve without compromise elsewhere. It is only by understanding the rules of the new contract that we can learn how to pursue a high income. It was Francis Bacon who said knowledge is power. Armed with the facts, we can succeed.

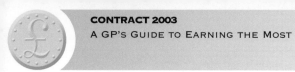

THE IDEAL PRACTICE

ETHOS

This book is concerned with wealth generation. So, when we come to look at the ideal practice, we are talking about the ideal practice for maximising profits. Certainly, there are many other ideals that can guide GPs in their everyday work: patient-centred focus, pleasant location, religious emphasis, academia, family-friendliness, team-based approach. The list is almost endless. Wealth generation does not disregard these other ideals – in fact, recognising what it is that makes a practice successful in other ways is one of the keys to unlocking a healthy financial future.

But if your practice is to be really profitable, then finances have to take a place up there with the other motivating forces. It is not good enough simply to expect the money to flow in for being a good doctor. The financial rewards of that policy are always mediocre.

High-earning practices make profitability one of their top priorities. They are not afraid to state the fact that their practice is a business, and the partners are effectively the shareholders. And, while the mission statement of the practice might be something along the lines of "To provide the highest quality medical care", there will always be the tacit aim of maximising profit alongside.

EXERCISE

A useful exercise is to sit down with your partners and try and decide how hard the practice wants to pursue a high income. Invariably, there will be as many opinions as there are partners, but it helps to reach common ground. The energetic pursuit of a shared vision is the first step towards success.

Write down what it is that each partner wants most of all to get out of being a doctor in your practice. Is it to have a high level of job satisfaction from providing excellent medical care? Is it to balance work and home life? Is it to follow their teaching/academic aims in life? Are there other doctors who want to achieve a high income?

Decide whether any of the chosen aims conflict with each other. Remember, high income and good quality medical care don't necessarily conflict, especially when considering the quality payments (see p. 75). Similarly, reducing stress by working shorter hours – say by ditching evening, weekend and night work – might pay dividends in terms of income if a partner is able to concentrate better on generating income elsewhere.

Try to draw a diagram of the forces that are pulling the doctors in different directions. Two examples are shown in Figure 1.

1:

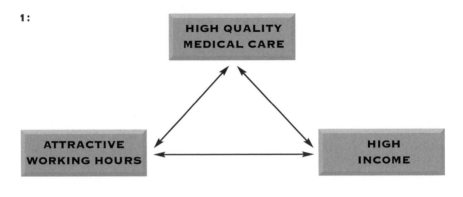

2:

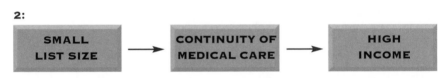

Figure 1. Two examples of forces pulling doctors in different directions.

In the first example, it is assumed that the triadic priorities for the partners are in conflict; that, for example, it is not possible to achieve high income and have plenty of time off. This may be so, or it might be possible to reach this state of affairs only by compromising patient care. For every change that the practice proposes, a decision will have to be made on where the partners are going to position themselves within their triangle.

The second example is a little simplistic, but has the advantage of driving in one direction. If the partners feel that the best way to earn a high income is to keep their list size small, to concentrate on reaching the highest quality targets for their patients, then they have a good model for future development of their practice.

Writing down the aims of the partners like this is a good way of exposing the different motivating forces within a practice. If different doctors have different views on which way the practice should be going, it is better that everyone is aware of those differences, rather than all pulling in opposite directions and unknowingly working against each other.

If there is a variety of opinion, then that can be seen as a strength in the practice. Differences of opinion can be discussed openly and can guide the overall aims and ambitions of the practice as a whole. Open and honest consideration of the other partners' views can influence individual bias and lead to common ground.

Having, hopefully, reached a joint position on the future financial direction the practice wishes to take, it is important to write something down. The statement of financial intent will be a guideline for the practice management, will focus staff and will guide future decision making by the partners.

EXAMPLE

The partners of the Crossroads Practice decided, after much lively discussion, that they would all like to earn more money but also to reduce stress levels by finishing work at 7 p.m. every day. They wrote this down as a statement of intent as part of their 5-year business plan, which was typed up by their practice manager.

The financial partner and the manager then sat down to look at the different sources of practice income and when the work for those sources was conducted. It appeared that most partners were struggling to fit in their private medicals late into the evening, after the end of evening surgery. Those that were continuing to work in the local out-of-hours co-operative were also finishing work late, at 11.30 p.m. Income from quality payments was low, as the practice was failing to meet the higher targets for most diseases.

It was decided that by dropping out-of-hours work and making the evening surgeries slightly later, time could be freed up in the afternoons for the partners to do private medicals before evening surgery. After discussion at the next partners meeting, all agreed that this would reduce stress levels, but concern was voiced about the loss of income from out-of-hours work. Calculations had shown that this loss could be more than compensated for if the higher quality targets were reached. It was agreed that the partners would each spend one evening a month conducting a chronic disease management clinic to boost quality payments, and that out-of-hours work would be dropped. Private medicals were given regular afternoon slots and, as a result, the practice successfully bid for a lucrative contract to provide medico-legal reports.

The ethos of the practice – to focus on income in a balanced, unanimous way – paid dividends.

PRACTICE STRUCTURE

The business structure of general practice has been run along traditional lines since the inception of the NHS in 1948. GMS practices have been run by the partners, who have also done the majority of the clinical work. Salaried doctors, whether registrars, assistants or locums, have made up a distinct minority of the medical workforce, and this model has been enforced by both the Medical Practices Committee's cap on GP Principal numbers and also by the old Red Book rules governing basic practice allowance.

The new contract for GMS practices changes all that. It is now entirely up to individual practices how they structure both the business management and medical workforce within their walls. It is no longer necessary to replace a retiring partner with an identical substitute in order to maintain practice income. Indeed, it is financially favourable to restrict the number of profit-sharing partners in order to maximise individual shares and to employ salaried doctors to help provide medical care.

With this in mind, partnerships are now faced with the challenging task of balancing the proportion of salaried doctors and partners within the practice, and aiming for list sizes that provide for optimum use of existing partners.

The ideal make-up of a GMS practice will be dictated by several factors.

- The availability of doctors in your area.

- The partners' preferences for providing management/specialisation/ out-of-hours.

- The skills of other employed staff.

- The management culture.

- Opportunities for work outside the practice.

- Competition with other local providers.

- Demographics of the local population.

Opportunities to change a practice's structure may only occur when an existing partner retires or resigns. If this is unlikely in the near future, then changing the practice list size may provide another way of bringing about major change to the balance of staff and partners.

The only other option is to consider merging or splitting partnerships. With some practices being in crisis over the shortage of applicants for partnership vacancies, this may be an attractive alternative.

EXERCISE

In order to design the ideal structure for your practice, it is a good idea to hold a free-flow, no-holds-barred thinking session in which established ideas are thrown out of the window. Start by imagining you have no patients, but that you are trying to set up a completely new practice in the same locality.

Decide what sort of practice you want to run. Do you, for example, want to do any out-of-hours or private work? Would you like a day off in the week? How important is it for you to achieve quality targets? Do you like the idea of specialising in cardiology, or vasectomies, or medical management? Can you write, or appear on the television, or teach?

What will new patients need in terms of access to services, number of appointments with a doctor or a nurse, private medicals, etc.? What degree of continuity of medical care will be appropriate to them? Is there much chronic disease in the area?

Look at the opportunities available in your area. Start with the patients themselves.
- Is there a large population of young men requesting vasectomy referral?
- Do many people ask for insurance medicals or BUPA-style check-ups?

Then look at surrounding practices.
- Are there any that have ditched out-of-hours work, closed their lists to new patients, or abandoned contraceptive/child health/screening work?

Move on to the Primary Care Organisation.
- Are they looking for someone to do a chest pain clinic, to visit local nursing homes, or sit on their management board?

And finally cast the net further.
- Is there work available providing insurance companies, solicitors or the police with medical skills?

All these opportunities are potential sources of income. Some are worth more than others from the financial point of view, but each has its own value to you from a non-financial angle as well. This will depend on your personal interests and skills, and here, again, you need to cast off any preconceived ideas about your abilities. It is possible to learn new skills as a GP. If you think there is a place for a GP in your area to set up a vasectomy service, then go and learn how to do vasectomies (see p. 43).

Having decided which services to provide, look at your practice as it is set up at the moment. Think about how you and your partners provide the NHS patients on your lists with medical care, and how private services are worked in. How far are you from the wish list you generated above?

Do any of the partners in your practice have the skills to provide any of the new services you identified? Is there a willingness to learn new skills? If not, then think how those skills might be brought into the practice – say, by employing a doctor or nurse on a sessional or salaried basis.

Are the premises adequate for the task in mind, and do the staff have the skills and time to help run the proposed services? These things can be changed. Don't let them stand in the way of progress, especially if there is a threat to future profitability.

This sort of lateral thinking is based on SCOT analysis (Strengths, Challenges, Opportunities and Threats) and should always feel a little far-fetched. It is only by shedding the restraints of the where-are-we-now that we can get to the where-do-we-want-to-be.

EXAMPLE

The partners of New Practice noticed they were referring about 20 patients a year to the local hospital 20 miles away for private vasectomies at a cost of £170 each. They assumed other practices in their area were doing the same and calculated that this was worth about £20,000 of business a year. They had never imagined they would end up doing vasectomies themselves, but decided to start up a clinic and poach the business among local patients by being cheaper and closer than the existing provider.

The partner with an interest in minor surgery contacted an out-of-area vasectomy clinic, who were more than happy to train him to do vasectomies. The practice nurses also went along to observe the procedure, make an inventory of the necessary surgical equipment, and learn about the counselling and paperwork side of things.

After several sessions of first observing and then being observed doing operations, the partner felt confident to start up in his own practice. His early patients were informed about the level of his training and offered the choice of either referral or in-house surgery. After several successful procedures the service was rolled out in full, charging local patients £140 and advertising the service to surrounding practices as well.

As demand for the service increased, the vasectomy partner started doing a clinic every 2 weeks instead of a surgery, while his clinical work was covered by the registrar. The overall profit to the practice was a little over £10,000 a year, after allowing for staff time and overheads.

INFORMATION TECHNOLOGY

The new GMS contract for general practice makes big demands on practices' IT systems. The quality payments, while based on trust reporting, demand the accurate recording of a great deal of clinical data in a retrievable format and this is only possible with advanced computer use.

Practices that are reluctant to embrace the ethos of detailed computer records are at a disadvantage, while those partnerships that still carry a doctor who doesn't use the computer at all are doomed to financial disaster. It is a sad fact that the only way to prove we are working well as doctors under the new contract is to make us dedicate more of our time to computers!

The detailed requirements of data selection are dealt with in the chapters on quality, but there are a few points to make on IT in general first. The three main suppliers of medical software used in general practice – Vision, EMIS and Torex – have all been caught short by the publication of the new GMS contract. Existing templates, searches, audits and computerised claims are still relevant only to the old Red Book. What is needed is a system designed with automatic search and claim facilities appropriate to the new GMS contract. Until computer suppliers are able to produce the software, we have to make do with what we have.

Primary Care Organisations (PCOs) are now responsible for 100% funding of practice computers. With this in mind, it is worth looking at ways to choose what to buy and, possibly, to switch systems. There are three areas of computerisation that directly affect income: recording quality data, retrieving quality data and electronic claims.

CLINICAL DATA RECORDING

The essential need for clinical IT systems is the ability to record data in a retrievable way. If, for example, you do a diabetes check on a patient, you must be able to record those aspects of the consultation that need to be counted in order to substantiate your claim for the appropriate level of quality payment. Furthermore, the software should be able to search all your records and produce a list of those patients in whom the level has been reached. Finally, recording and retrieving data in this way must be quick and easy – doing the medicine is hard enough, without the computer slowing things up!

Vision, EMIS and Torex all now operate templates to record data for many diseases.

Existing templates may have gaps, for example Vision not having the means to record quantitative values for 24-hour ambulatory blood pressure results. (This problem can be circumvented by recording a numerical value under Read code 246Z for "Blood pressure reading". While not strictly clinically accurate, at least a retrievable record of blood pressure is made, helping achieve a higher target.)

The three main computer suppliers have promised to produce templates for all 10 clinical quality areas. These will be supplied as upgrades in the usual way and, in most cases, be available as downloadable patches via practices' NHSnet connections. In the meantime, new templates can be custom built within all three systems (see Appendix 1). Customising templates is strongly recommended. The main advantages of designing your own templates are:

- An exact match between what the contract demands and what you record.

- Personalisation to encourage the use of templates.

- Insertion of templates within convenient screen layout.

- Flexibility to alter the template in future, if necessary.

Learning how to design and customise templates requires a bit of time and effort, and should involve a computer-competent member of staff as well as the GPs. Everyone should jot down what they want recorded on the template for each disease. Remember to make sure you have covered all those areas required to reach the top quality levels. Don't include unnecessary data, i.e. data that will not need to be recovered on all patients for clinical or financial purposes.

Having agreed the list, put the items for inclusion in a sensible order, grouping together similar items, e.g. blood test results, then height and weight, lifestyle factors and examination findings. Use the Read codes for each item as specified in the chapter on Quality (see p. 75).

Using the template editing facility, known as the Wizard on most systems, construct a layout of the above Read-coded items, think up a suitable title, and paste the template into the system. Templates can be triggered to appear on screen when selected Read codes are entered during a normal consultation. Furthermore, if you are doing a specific clinic, say for diabetes, the computer can be set to display the diabetes template at the start of each new consultation.

For detailed instruction on exactly how to customise templates on your computer system, consult the manual or, better still, arrange for a trainer from the medical software company to come to the practice and show you how it's done (see Appendix 1).

MANAGER'S TIP

It is worth investing in good quality training. Train key personnel, including a doctor and a nurse. Give them protected time for their training. If you can afford it, spread the training over a couple of days about a week apart. This gives people a chance to try things and discover what they really learnt on the first session. Remember this is an investment that will pay dividends later.

AUDIT

If the practice has been using templates to record clinical data, then searches and audits should record accurate results easily. All three main medical software suppliers have advanced audit facilities available to search your data and record levels of achievement.

Customised searches are also easier to set up, following the Read codes used in the disease templates.

Quite often, however, the results of searches produce some surprises. For example, one system contains an automatic search on angina patients that only counts aspirin if it is prescribed as an anti-platelet drug, not if it is prescribed as a non-opioid analgesic. While this is clinically accurate, it is very misleading. The default when prescribing aspirin on this system is for it to be entered as an analgesic, so requiring the doctor to perform two or three extra mouse clicks to enter the right category. Unless the doctors know this they won't necessarily change category, and even if they do know, they might not feel inclined to do the extra work just for the sake of improving the audit!

To get round the problem it is essential to set up a customised search. This way the angina patients' records can be counted if they have aspirin on repeat prescription under either category and in any formulation. Furthermore, patients can be counted if they are on warfarin, dipyridamole or clopidogrel instead of aspirin, and those patients who buy their own aspirin can also be counted if they have a code for aspirin prophylaxis on their record.

Having set up the data entry templates in-house, a practice will have the knowledge to define its own searches to match. It is the knowledge of the data you want to retrieve that should dictate the content of the templates.

See Appendix 1 for details of how to gain the information needed in order to run detailed searches and audits.

Electronic claims

Under the old Red Book, computer systems had been set up to file Items of Service and Registration claims electronically. The Primary Care Agencies (PCAs) were able to process these claims, theoretically speeding up the process of paying practices, improving accuracy and reducing paperwork.

The new GMS contract has become operational ahead of the PCAs' ability to process claims electronically. Verification of the practices' success in achieving quality targets can be done by printing off a hard copy of the audit results and sending it to the PCO for payment.

Clearly, it will be to the financial advantage of practices if they are able to connect up to electronic claims. One word of warning, though. Always have a system for reconciling claims made and payments received. If you have done all the hard work to achieve a set target in the quality areas, don't let the PCA reject your claim. Reconciling claims is usually done by a system separate from the medical system. Keep a log of all electronic payments applied for, noting the date sent and the dates the clinical work was conducted. Cross-check on receipt of payment authorisation that all eligible fees have been agreed by the PCA, and check again when the quarterly returns are received at the practice, noting the actual money transferred. This work can be done by the practice manager or a member of staff using a simple Excel-type spreadsheet. Claims made can be totalled monthly and downloaded into Excel from most medical systems.

Accountancy

Using a good firm of accountants will more than pay for itself in enhanced profits to a practice. Many medical accountants already provide their clients with a very high quality of service in the following areas.

- Preparation of partnership tax returns.

- Defining partnership shares.

- Maximising personal professional costs to offset against tax.

There are other areas of accountancy expertise that can, and should, be required by the practice in order to maximise overall profit. These cover:

- The day-to-day running of the business records of the practice.

- Planning for major change or investment.

- Proactively advising practices on forthcoming legislation or opportunities.

- Advising practices of their financial performance.

- Comparisons with other practices' performance.

- Remedies for under-performance.

Most accountancy firms will be able to supply these requirements, especially if they have a partner who specialises in medical practices. It is, however, necessary to ask for this level of service. Furthermore, the onus is on the practice to advise their accountant in good time of major plans for change.

EXAMPLE

The Village Practice had always had their annual accounts and tax return completed for them by the local branch of a small accountancy firm. This had been perfectly adequate for many years, but the partners decided they needed specialist advice on how to improve profitability under the new GMS contract. Despite meeting with their accountant and asking him for advice on the best way to change things for the better, the advice they received was vague and confusing, and seemed to relate to the old Red Book system of payments.

When the partners were given the opportunity to move into new premises they felt the time had come to seek really good, expert, specialist accountancy help. After meeting with three accountants from different companies and getting quotes, they chose a firm of widely known specialists in the medical field and changed to the new firm.

A period of "orientation" meetings took place, whereby the accountant familiarised himself with his new clients. It was clear to him that their first priority was to improve their monitoring procedures for the quality payments by investing in a better computer system. This would maximise income from current work. Their next need was to have advice on the preparation of a business case for an application to the PCO for premises development.

His suggestions were met with relief by the partners, who had longed for this kind of specialist help. Furthermore, the accountant was able to compare the practice's financial performance with that of his many other clients and reassure them that they were actually slightly above average for overall profitability, staffing and private income. He was able to give the practice an accurate estimate of their likely profits should they choose to go into PMS, also by comparison with other practices on his books that had already taken the decision to change contracts.

After 2 years under new accountancy procedures, the practice had increased profits by 12%, more than covering the increased fees charged by the accountant.

Other areas of expert advice accountants should be expected to provide GPs with include:

- Tax planning.

- Formation of companies or partnerships with spouses to minimise tax liabilities.

- Premises planning.

- Superannuation and pension planning for partners and staff.

- Retirement and recruitment issues.

- Partnership splits and mergers.

- Computers.

- Practice management.

As well as receiving good, proactive advice from an accountant, GPs should also expect:

- Prompt responses to queries.

- Accounts prepared in good time, and certainly well ahead of the tax deadlines.

- Accounts presented in a format useful as a management tool.

- A named contact within the accountancy firm.

- E-mail for quick answers to questions.

- Accurate estimates of cost of accountancy.

- Value for money.

If practices find themselves dissatisfied with the level of service they currently receive, then serious consideration should be given to putting out a tender. Interview, say, three firms, including the present accountant, having written out a list of requirements as above.

A good source of information on accountancy firms can be obtained from AISMA, the Association of Independent Specialist Medical Accountants:

48 St Leonards Road
Bexhill on Sea
East Sussex
TN40 1JB

Tel.: 01424 730345
Fax: 01424 730330
E-mail: aisma@honeybarrett.co.uk
www.aisma.org.uk

Specialist accountancy advice will appear to be more expensive, on the surface, than non-specialist advice. If you are satisfied with the practice's profits and don't see the point in rocking the boat, then stick with the accountant you have. But be prepared for your income to be eroded over the years compared to other GPs in your area and around the country. If, on the other hand, you are excited by the idea of improving the quality of the financial management of the practice and maximising your profits, then consider whether you have the right accountant for the job. A few thousand pounds spent on good advice can be returned to the practice within a few months through improved profitability.

ACCOUNTANT'S TIP

Certifying NHS profits for superannuation purposes is an area of specialised medical accountancy. For practices that keep private income and personal expenses outside of the partnership accounts, it is best to allocate as much of the expenses element as possible to non-GMS and private earnings. This will maximise NHS pensionable earnings.

BUSINESS PLANNING

There are companies of independent management consultants that offer to help GPs with business planning. They can be very expensive (over £1000 a day) and value for money is not always guaranteed. Having said that, there are situations in which it can be a wise move enlisting the help of an expert.

- Partnership splits.

- Practice mergers.

- Dismissing senior staff.

- Switching NHS contract to Personal Medical Services (PMS).

- Embarking on a new building project.

- Applying for dispensing rights.

These major upheavals should affect a GP only once in a lifetime at the most. There are several reasons for enlisting the help of a qualified management consultant, most of which revolve around the lack of ability and knowledge on the part of doctors.

- Detailed appreciation of legal matters, e.g. employment law.

- Knowledge of specialist field, e.g. dispensing.

- Objective approach to problems.

- Comparison with other practices.

- Negotiating and chairing skills.

- Networking with outside stakeholders/advisers.

- Dedication to task – no clinical commitments.

- Time to write up, analyse and report to partners.

- Structured approach to follow-up.

While the above examples of major change should occur infrequently, it is a good idea to get into the habit of regular (say, annual) business planning meetings without the help of an outside management consultant. These meetings usually take at least half a day and should involve all the partners and the practice manager. The aim should be to adjust the direction and overall aims of the business side of the practice.

Find a suitable venue, which may not necessarily be the practice premises, organise locum cover and book lunch. Before the day, write out a list of aims and objectives, based on short-, medium- and long-term goals. They may include:

- Solving the lack of suitable practice premises.

- Improving profitability.

- Hitting top quality targets.

- Motivating staff and management.

- Dealing with impending retirement of a partner.

- Diversifying services.

- Looking for new markets/advertising.

- Improving the computer system of the practice.

- Reducing time wastage.

- Managing out-of-hours work.

Issues of this magnitude are generally too big to fit into the routine weekly practice meeting of 1 or 2 hours. They deserve special attention in an environment free of interruptions. No special skills are required other than the sort of detailed personal knowledge of the practice that all partners and managers have. It is, however, essential to be disciplined in the execution of the day, so that time is not wasted with sidetracks and waffle. Partner time is expensive, so results are needed.

Having defined the aims of the day, decide who will take minutes at the meeting. This is usually the practice manager, unless the partners are meeting alone to discuss problems with the management, in which case a partner should be nominated. A chairman should be elected and an agenda produced, listing the time to be allocated to each item.

PITFALL

One of the problems with having no outside help on such occasions is the tendency to tunnel vision. While working with a problem in the everyday grind of surgeries, visits and paperwork, doctors can make hasty, ill-thought-out decisions on how they would solve the problem themselves. Latching on to their solution, and letting it ferment for several days or weeks in the run-up to a business meeting, can lead them to an entrenched position from which they are reluctant to be prised.

Recognising this, encourage your partners to approach problem-solving from a new angle. Listen to each other's views first, reappraise the problem by looking at it from someone else's viewpoint, think how someone else might solve it and finally try to steer the partnership towards a unified solution. Fashionably known as "thinking outside the box", this lateral approach is much more likely to produce consensus and unity than to lead to division and strife.

Next steps

Ideally, the practice that is striving to join the elite band of highest-earning practices should look at profitability early on in their business planning cycle. Having already decided to make profits a priority under the new contract, what is the next step?

Start by looking at the opportunities for income generation and cost-cutting under the new contract. Going through the contract section by section will be necessary in order to avoid missing anything. Referral to the chapters on Practice Size and Out-of-Hours will help highlight those areas most likely to affect profits. Opportunities for earning non-GMS health service income should also be looked at (see chapter on Diversity). Private earnings possibilities should be explored, both from NHS patients and outside patients (see page 35).

In the ideal practice, the partners are not afraid to challenge commonly held beliefs, including their own. In analysing their situation, they should not be reluctant to explore the weaknesses of the practice, both medical and managerial. Threats to future financial success should be fully and openly explored.

EXAMPLE

The partners of The Friendly Practice had had the same manager for many years and developed strong personal ties and a sense of loyalty to their team. Sadly the manager, who had risen through the ranks of practice reception work, lacked the skills needed to move the practice forward. There was a tacit understanding that a new manager was needed but, whenever this was alluded to, a frisson of anxiety spread among the partners, who were reluctant to upset what had been a successful team for so long. A business meeting was held by the partners. Discussion revealed that all the doctors felt the same and that there was a lack of knowledge about how to change practice managers correctly. It was decided to ask a management consultancy to help. The partners were helped to see that the problem needed to be tackled and that they could not tackle it alone. This uncomfortable but brave process helped the partners to formulate a more cohesive financial plan for the future and resulted in the appointment of a high-calibre specialist practice manager.

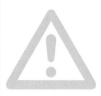

WORKING PRACTICES

The key points that, together, summarise the best way a practice will maximise its profits are:

- Practices with top-rate databases on their patients and treatments.

- Proactive rather than reactive teams.

- Good management of time.

- Well-organised GPs with strong staff teams and good skills mix among them.

- Those with the most competent and skilled practice managers.

- GPs who plan ahead, are forward-looking and work together.

- Stable partnerships.

- Close involvement with the PCO.

Financial disaster can be expected to befall:

- Practices involved in partnership disputes.

- GPs with inadequate resources, such as staff, equipment and space.

- Doctors with excessive numbers of patients.

- Those without the necessary data available on their patients.

- Badly organised practices.

- Bad managers of time.

DIVERSITY

For most GPs, the greater part of practice income is generated by NHS fees from their main contract, whether GMS or PMS. For the highest earning practices, maximising those fees must take top priority.

Looking at those few practices in the top 2% of the earnings range, however, it is clear that other earnings feature heavily, and this is why it pays to diversify. So long as you can be certain that NHS fees have been maximised, it is a good idea to focus on non-contract NHS income and private work if earnings are to reach their true potential.

Apart from boosting profits, other advantages of diversity are:

- The flexibility to increase or decrease workload to suit the practice.

- The development of areas of specialist interest.

- Protection against future poor NHS pay awards.

- Networking outside the practice.

- Establishing an escape route from general practice (change of career).

- Tax benefits of incorporation for private earnings.

- Private pensions for spouses.

Some of the opportunities for diversification from core NHS work are dictated by local needs; setting up as a police surgeon, for example, will only be possible if the local force has a vacancy. However, many of the opportunities are national and there is a shortage of GPs willing to take on the work. Examples include:

- Medico-legal examination and reporting.

- Drug company research.

- Occupational health.

- Sports medicine.

- Benefits agency work.

- Medical writing.

- Primary Care Organisation (PCO) board work.

- Out-of-hours work for co-operatives, deputising services and PCOs.

- Additional services for non-provider practices, e.g. family planning.

- Enhanced services work for PCO initiatives, e.g. specialist clinics.

- Medical work for hospital trusts.

- Medical education.

The level of pay for these varies enormously, with some of the most rewarding being the least well remunerated! Obviously, all we have learnt about cost-benefit analysis will have to be applied before leaping into any contract. Consider carefully the knock-on effect of taking up valuable doctor time and the potential loss of income from other sources, not least the core NHS fees.

Other private income can be generated within existing practices, but involves delegating tasks to other members of staff. Travel vaccines, private blood tests, research contracts and some occupational health work can be delegated to practice nurses. So long as the priorities are to focus on high-yield, low-overhead contracts then profitability can be maintained, even if extra nursing hours have to be paid for. Other practice staff can generate private income from tasks such as data collection for research and marketing, drug company information, management consultancy and teaching. Seek out this work by maintaining an active network of links to outside stakeholders to the practice: the PCO, the local academic departments and drug companies. Market your practice actively and exploit all the resources you have.

For big contracts, such as some occupational health and drug company work, it will almost certainly be necessary to increase staff time, either nursing or medical, to fulfil both the private contract requirements and the core practice work. This can be managed successfully with proper planning and can result in both a boost to practice profits and little effect on practice manpower.

EXAMPLE

A large multinational drug company approached the Pound Lane Practice asking if they would be interested in participating in a post-marketing exercise. The work involved interviewing patients, measuring blood pressures and sending blood to the company for analysis. Apart from the practice's own patients, there would be many more from the surrounding area. The estimated numbers were somewhere between 200 and 300 patients for a single check-up each, spread over the course of a year.

The payments were to be made per capita and were equal to £25 per patient. With income possibly as high as £7500, the practice felt there was a good margin, even after increasing the practice nurse's hours by 1 hour per week to accommodate the work.

One of the ways to improve the profitability of private work is to fit it in around existing timetables and use the existing facilities of the practice. This is most useful for small volume, intermittent work.

Medico-legal reports, which can attract up to £200 for half an hour's work, are a good example. These can be fitted in around GMS work and involve virtually no expenditure. A glance at the classified advertisement section of the BMJ or Doctor magazine usually reveals a handful of private companies trying to recruit GPs for this work. The majority of cases are very simple whiplash injuries following minor car accidents and giving an opinion is not difficult. In order to ensure you get plenty of work from these companies, send them an example of a well-presented medical report (patient identifiers omitted). Use high-quality paper, double-spaced type and lots of sub-headings. Include a CV and copies of your registration and medical indemnity certificates. Promise to provide reports within 7 days and offer appointments on at least 3 days a week. Once you have had you first report accepted, make it into a template in Word and use macros to enter new patient details for subsequent reports. This cuts preparation time in half and almost doubles the profit margin on this type of private work.

For an example of this type of medico-legal report, refer to Appendix 2. Notice that some of the wording of the report is a legal requirement following Lord Woolf's recommendations to the legal profession (highlighted in italics in the Appendix).

OVERCOMING INERTIA

Choosing to take on extra work might seem bonkers to GPs who feel under pressure already. The immediate feeling is "How can I do any more than I am doing at the moment?" Indeed, most people's workload fills the time available to it, creating a feeling of working to maximum capacity.

The new contract opens up new areas of potential income generation from opting to provide more services, whether they are specialist GP roles such as endoscopy or minor surgery, or providing GMS services to other practices that have opted out of, say, out-of-hours or maternity.

Practices that have decided to maximise income need not be held back by partners who feel they cannot work any harder. There are ways improving profitability while maintaining, or even reducing, existing workload patterns.

The first task is to establish your hourly rate of pay. Take the total number of hours worked in an average month, and compare this with your total income. This tells you the average rate of pay for all the work you do and will help you to decide whether new work is worth more.

For example:

$$\text{Surgeries, visits and paperwork} = 200 \text{ hours}$$
$$\text{Saturday morning once a month} = 3$$
$$\text{Co-operative shifts} = 22$$
$$\text{Private work} = 6$$
$$\text{Work from home} = 4$$
$$\text{Total} = 235$$
$$1/12 \text{ of total annual gross profit (say £60k)} = \textbf{5000}$$

$$\text{Hourly rate} = \textbf{£21.30}$$

This is how much you earn from all your work, averaged out, and can be used to quantify the value of new work by comparison. Do not confuse this with the rate you should charge for your time when submitting a bid for new work, or an invoice for work done. That rate is very much higher.

When assessing the profitability of new work it is essential to know the true cost of providing that work. For example, look at doing a clinical assistantship at a local hospital. If a partner is taken away from the surgery to do this, how will that absent partner's practice work be done ? Can the remaining partners cover, or will a locum or assistant have to be found ? The cost of providing cross-cover should be added into the equation used to calculate the profitability of the new work. Partners cost £21.30 per hour in the above example. Locums are considerably more expensive. If the income minus the costs does not exceed your current hourly rate, then the work is not financially worthwhile.

If there is a lot of new work available, and this may be the case in your area under the new GMS contract, then it might be worthwhile considering taking on a salaried assistant. The sudden leap in costs of doing this can be a difficult blow to profits initially, but the time freed up as a result can generate huge opportunities for partners to take on new income-generating roles. This can be seen not as extra work, but as alternative work; partners are happy and profits can rise as well.

Diversification can also apply to the use of practice premises. Your surgery building can generate considerable private income for very little effort. Subletting rooms to private and complementary practitioners involves some work initially, but thereafter it's money for old rope. One word of caution, however; under the present GMS contract, notional rent reimbursement can be withdrawn if private income exceeds 10% of total GMS. This is very difficult for primary care agencies to police and one of the ways around the problem is to charge private users a large service fee instead of rent. The figures can be about the same, but an itemised breakdown of the costs of running the practice, apportioned to the private user, should negate any breach of the rent rules.

RESPONSIBILITY FOR INCOME GENERATION

All partners in an ideal practice should share the feeling of responsibility for income generation. New opportunities for lucrative work don't always present themselves to the person best able to take advantage of them, but the practice in which everyone is "on the lookout" for new openings is the one that will prosper most. Furthermore, if all the partners share in the express aim of generating income as a priority for the practice, then that aim is more likely to be achieved.

Within the overall brief of improving the finances of the practice, there are specific roles that are best divided up among the partners. Detailed knowledge of how best to maximise income within an area can be developed by the partner, who then reports back to the others on a regular basis.

For a practice under the new GMS contract, the areas are:

- Finances and accounts.

- Personnel and training.

- Premises.

- Clinical quality.

- Organisational quality.

- Additional services.

- Enhanced services.

- Prescribing and dispensing.

- Primary Health Care Team (PHCT)/PCO liaison.

- Private work.

Before any of the partners set off in pursuit of their allotted tasks, it should be decided who is the best person for each job. Responsibility for overall practice finances and accounting should be given to the partner with knowledge of accounting principles, authority and skills in the development and implementation of partnership strategy. They should be assisted by the practice manager and accountant, and should have protected time for this aspect of their work.

Personnel and training should be given to the partner who is good at people management: interviewing, sizing up personalities, dispute resolution, employment law, motivating and rewarding.

Premises should be the responsibility of the practice manager, inasmuch as the established building will effectively run itself. A partner should be allocated to the role, however, to oversee value for money, new uses and opportunities, premises development/extension, branch surgery development and subletting.

The 10 clinical quality areas (see page 82) should ideally be divided up among the partners, as they each demand a great deal of organisational setting up, monitoring, audit, reporting and improving. Sharing them out helps all partners to appreciate the importance of being guided by others on how best to record clinical data for the financial benefit of the practice. One partner, however, should bear overall responsibility for clinical quality, and they should have skills in managing computer data entry and extraction and in compiling reports.

Organisational quality should be the responsibility of the practice manager, with the help of a partner who has skills in change management and an eye for detail and monitoring; in other words, a well-organised, methodical person with a knowledge of payment procedures.

Dispensing is a sizeable specialisation. A single partner should have responsibility for this area, in conjunction with the dispensary manager or practice manager, and have protected time for monitoring formularies, negotiating drug company deals and running "the shop".

Private work is to be encouraged by every partner, should be actively sought by all and ideally be part of the everyday work of the partnership. It helps to have one partner nominated in charge, if only that they may have knowledge of setting up contracts, negotiating rates and an established network beyond the practice with which to cast a wide net in the trawl for new opportunities.

PROTECTED TIME

The reasons why the partners should manage general practice are twofold. First they have a unique insight into the mechanisms of doing the work that attracts the money, and secondly they have a vested interest in getting it right.

Being involved is as much about getting your hands dirty in the small print of pounds and pence, as it is about delegating tasks correctly. The partner who spends hours every month poring over the details of his partners' consultations looking for missed claims is not only a sad person; he is wasting expensive partner time that should be delegated to someone else.

Negotiating useful systems for maximising income is an organisational role. It demands vision, lateral thinking, detailed knowledge of working mechanisms, checking and teamwork. Protected time is needed for this work to take place effectively. Sometimes the time needed is as a one-off – for example, interviewing a new member of staff. Other tasks are more complex and demand a regular session, such as running a dispensary or building new premises.

Giving partners protected time for management not only enables the job to be done more effectively; it conveys a sense of value to the work. The cost to the practice can be measured, and the gains must outweigh those costs. Half a day spent away from the patients on practice management, at a cost of several hundred pounds to the practice, must reap rewards above and beyond that if it is to be repeated. There is nothing quite like this notion for ensuring partners make best use of their time.

POTENTIAL INCOME

The new GMS contract is still in its infancy and, accordingly, examples of maximum incomes are yet to emerge. Practices that have traditionally been among the highest earning, however, will be aiming to maximise income from all sources, both GMS and private.

Assuming this is your aim, what are the implications for striving to achieve the top? Financial modelling can help predict future profits in general practice based on traditional levels of achievement and calculations based on the new contract fees.

Let's assume you have decided to keep your commitment to out-of-hours for now, to continue to provide the widest possible range of traditional general practice services, to achieve the maximum quality target in all areas and to take up some of the enhanced services work on offer from the local PCO. Let's also assume that you are able to achieve all this without losing any of the private income you previously enjoyed.

Sums of £120,000 annual gross profit per partner will be achievable in mixed NHS/private practices providing the full range of services over the next 3 years.

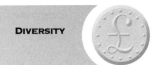

DIVERSITY

GMS — THE RANGE OF SERVICES

GMS practices provide services to the NHS under three broad areas.

- Essential services.

- Additional services.

- Enhanced services.

ESSENTIAL SERVICES

These cover:

1. Management of patients who are ill or believe themselves to be ill, with conditions from which recovery is generally expected, for the duration of that condition, including relevant health promotion advice and referral as appropriate, reflecting patient choice wherever practicable.

2. General management of patients who are terminally ill.

3. Management of chronic disease in the manner determined by the practice, in discussion with the patient.

All practices being paid under a GMS contract must provide these services between the hours of 8.00 a.m. and 6.30 p.m., Monday to Friday, from their practice premises and elsewhere within their practice area (usually the patient's home) if that is clinically appropriate, as decided by the GP.

The payment for this work is included in the practice's global sum, as calculated from the Carr–Hill allocation formula. This formula takes account of the number of patients, their age and sex, their morbidity and mortality, nursing/residential home status, list turnover, rurality and staff costs.

Practices whose global sum is lower than expected, due to underweighting, can opt to be paid via the Minimum Practice Income Guarantee (MPIG). This sum is based on historical earnings under the Red Book and is calculated by the local Primary Care Agency.

Either way, there is little the GP can do to maximise the payment for essential services. The amount is set by a predetermined formula for a set practice. However, there is an economy of scale within the Carr–Hill formula that acts as a disincentive for small practices. Increases in the global sum can be achieved by attracting more patients to the practice, especially if they are in rural areas or nursing/residential homes. So long as there is no corresponding increase in practice costs as a result, and while the extra medical manpower can be provided by salaried doctors, it is possible to increase practice profitability by getting larger. The same ends can be achieved by merging practices and rationalising the practice staff, and also by taking over the list of a neighbouring practice (e.g. on retirement of a single-hander).

ADDITIONAL SERVICES

These cover:

1. Cervical screening.

2. Contraceptive services.

3. Childhood immunisations.

4. Other immunisations (e.g. tetanus) excluding influenza.

5. Child health surveillance.

6. Antenatal and postnatal care.

7. Basic minor surgery (curettage, cautery and cryocautery of warts, verrucae and other skin lesions).

8. Out-of-hours care, until April 2004 (no opt-out guaranteed until December 2004).

Most GMS practices are expected to provide these services unless there are special circumstances (e.g. inability to recruit GPs to the practice). The payment for additional services is included in the global sum. Opting out of these services will reduce the global sum by the average values shown in Table 1.

Additional service	Opt-out price for 2004/2005 (indicative £ per GP)	Opt-out price for 2005/2006 (indicative £ per GP)	Percentage of global sum
Cervical screening	1203	1221	1.1
Child health surveillance	758	769	0.7
Minor surgery	654	663	0.6
Maternity medical services	2296	2330	2.1
Contraceptive services	2658	2698	2.4
Childhood immunisations and pre-school booster	1059	1075	1.0
Other immunisations	2220	2253	2.0
Out-of-hours	6000	6000	5.5

Table 1. Opt-out prices and percentage of global sum for additional services

The income lost to the practice as a result of opting out of all these services would be considerable. As practice staff perform the majority of all but the out-of-hours, practices still stand to gain considerable profit by providing these services. Opting out of out-of-hours is dealt with on page 68. If a practice really is struggling to provide the manpower to fulfil its additional services commitments, consider contracting the service out. A neighbouring practice may be willing to do the extra work for less than the opt-out price, especially if they are convinced by the economies of scale argument. Put a proposal to them. Alternatively, consider buying in the services of a family planning provider, the local midwifery service or a community paediatrics service.

If yours is the practice that is successfully able to perform the full range of additional services with ease, look around to see if you can take on extra work in this field. Either contract yourselves direct to the practices opting out or go to the PCO and offer to provide the extra services as a local enhanced service.

ENHANCED SERVICES (SEE PAGE 109)

There are three types of enhanced service: directed, national and local.

Directed enhanced services

These are extra services that are outside the remit of essential and additional services, that the PCO must provide and that have a nationally negotiated specification and price. They include: provision for seeing violent patients, improved access, childhood immunisation targets, influenza immunisation, quality information preparation and advanced minor surgery (above simple cautery for skin lesions).

Practices will already have considerable expertise and infrastructure to provide many of these services. Have a close dialogue with your PCO about which services you can offer to them, not only for your patients but for those of other practices. These services are entirely voluntary and there may be doctors in your area who would rather not try to provide them.

National enhanced services

These are like directed enhanced services in that their specification and price are negotiated nationally, but unlike directed services they are not mandatory for PCOs. These services may have been provided by secondary care or other providers within the NHS or social services. Examples include: intra-partum care, anticoagulant monitoring, IUCD fitting, drug and alcohol misuse services, specialised sexual health services, specialised depression services, multiple sclerosis services, enhanced care of the homeless, immediate care and first response care, near-patient testing and minor injury services.

If your practice currently provides these services, make sure you get the opportunity to be paid for them via a national enhanced services contract. Doctors in rural and remote areas will be asked by their PCO to continue to provide services in this way. If you don't currently provide these services, look at the service specifications to see if you could provide the services at a profit. Remember, you can buy in the medical/nursing expertise to provide the work and use the practice simply as an administrative tool and contract-holder.

Local enhanced services

These are extra services that practices may provide that are outside the remit of essential and additional services, and that are negotiated locally between the practice and the PCO. They may include such things as: cover for a local cottage hospital, the provision of additional services to an opted-out practice, running an adolescent health clinic at a local school or continuing to provide Saturday morning surgeries after December 2004.

If you are already providing these services, make sure you tell your PCO. Work out how much it costs you to provide the service, and decide whether you want to continue to provide the service or not. Fixing the price is by negotiation with the PCO, but their need for you to continue doing the work will dictate how hard you can drive up the price. If there is no alternative provider you should take a hard line. Don't listen to their pleas for clemency, and certainly don't agree to do the work "to help out the NHS". Remember, enhanced services are optional under the GMS contract. If the price is not appealing, just say no!

PRIVATE WORK

In an earlier chapter we mentioned that one of the values of diversifying was the protection against financial under-performance in any one area of work. The main GMS contract might fail to bring in the expected financial rewards for several reasons.

- Missed quality targets.

- Local competition from other providers.

- Limited range of services due to understaffing.

- Inability to limit workload.

- Poorly negotiated national and local pay settlements.

- Desire to abandon out-of-hours.

- Under-utilisation of the computer.

- Failure to chase up NHS payments.

- Low level of payment for work done, e.g. treating violent patients.

In the thriving and successful GP practice there is a diversity of private work, sometimes accounting for up to 50% of practice income, and any practice wanting to maximise profits should certainly be doing some private work.

ACCOUNTANT'S TIP

In the year 2000, the average GP's non-GMS/PMS income was £16,097. High non-GMS earnings were a significant feature of the highest earning GPs in the UK.

Some examples of the private work of a GP are:

- Acupuncture.

- Authorship.

- Benefits agency work.

- Committee fees, e.g. BMA/MDU/RCGP/LMC.

- Directorships, e.g. co-operative/ambulance trust.

- Drug company research/trials/adviser.

- Expert witness.

- Hospice work.

- Hospital work.

- Independent tribunal service.

- Medical audit advisory group work.

- Medical research ethics committee.

- Occupational health.

- PCO board/meetings.

- Pilots' licences.

- Police surgeon.

- Retainer, e.g. nursing homes/private schools/MoD.

- Review panel – disciplinary.

- Sports medicine.

- Summative assessments.

- Travel clinic.

- Training/teaching.

INSURANCE MEDICALS

Traditionally, NHS general practices have attracted private fees for doing medicals and insurance (PMA) reports. The fees for this work are relatively good, but the volume is controlled by patient and insurance company demand. Consequently, income from this source is usually limited to £2000–3000 a year per doctor.

This figure can be increased. Just think how few insurance medicals you do compared with the number of PMA reports. Who is doing the medical if you're not? The answer is that the insurance companies are asking private agencies of doctors and nurses to provide the medical examinations for them. The private agencies pay their doctors slightly less, but guarantee them a certain volume of work, which means the doctors earn more than they would through direct insurance company requests. The agencies make their financial profit by charging the insurance companies slightly more per medical. Finally, the insurance companies benefit by having their medicals completed to agreed standards of quality, turnaround time, cost and volume. Also, it is more cost-effective for the insurance companies to liaise with one or two agencies than hundreds of individual doctors.

This is the competition. In the free market economy, this is what you're up against. Whenever you do a PMA report or insurance medical, send the company a covering letter expressing an interest in providing a medical examinations service for them. Make sure the medical form you do is completed fully, accurately, promptly and legibly. Offer to do the medicals within a short turnaround time and extol the virtues of your experience and the facilities available to you, including peak flow, ECG, blood testing, spirometry, audiology and anything else you have. Play up your service. Offer pre-test counselling for HIV tests. Confirm that you are willing to complete the examination for the agreed BMA rate (which will be cheaper for the company than using an agency). Say that you have the capacity to do medicals not only on your own patients, but on patients of other doctors in the area and beyond. Only offer to do medicals in patients' homes if you are really sure the profits are worth it. In my experience, travelling time makes this a non-starter. Using this mildly predatory approach will increase the number of requests you get by poaching work from the agencies.

When a request for a medical comes in, the instructing letter usually says that the patient has been asked to contact you to make an appointment. Don't wait for this to happen; ring the patient yourself and book them in before they change their mind. Make appointment times available outside office hours – the majority of applicants for this type of medical are in work. Make sure you do the work on time and well. Develop a name for providing those companies that use you with a good service. You can then use this reputation to market yourself to other companies.

MEDICO-LEGAL REPORTS

A lucrative market for GPs services is emerging in the legal world. There is an increasing number of solicitors offering to represent people who have been injured in car accidents, and they inevitably need a doctor to give an opinion. In cases where the injuries are significant, the opinion of a specialist is required, but there are many minor cases where the only injury is whiplash. It is not necessary to have a detailed knowledge of spinal orthopaedics to examine the back and give an opinion on the findings in these cases.

Start by looking in the small ads section at the back of the BMJ or the free GP magazines such as *Doctor*. There are usually a handful of companies that manage the interface between solicitors and doctors, and their adverts aim to attract the attention of GPs for medico-legal work. They usually pay between £90 and £120 for examination and report, plus an hourly rate of £50–60 for going through the patient's medical records. With most straightforward cases of whiplash, the whole process can be completed in 30 minutes, delivering a return of about £250 per hour pro rata – very lucrative indeed. There are no overheads so, apart from doctor time, this is all profit.

If you approach one of these companies it is important to establish exactly how they wish the medical report to be presented. They should send you a list of headings of areas they want to be covered, which is usually based on:

- Patient details.

- Accident details.

- Injuries sustained.

- Psychological effects on the patient.

- Chronological progression of symptoms.

- Treatment.

- Past medical history.

- Loss as a result of accident.

- Examination findings.

- Present situation.

- Reasonableness (e.g. of amount of time off work).

- Prognosis.

- Recommendations (e.g. for further treatment).

- Summary.

Make sure you match their required format, e.g. double spacing, 90gsm paper, two copies, etc. There are certain statements that need to be included in the report to fulfil Lord Woolf's recommendations on giving evidence to the courts. These include:

- That the report is accurate to the best of your knowledge.

- That your opinion is given to the court, not to the patient's solicitor.

- That your opinion is not influenced by your responsibilities to the patient or the person paying for the report.

For an example of a medico-legal report, see Appendix 2.

Once you have established how to do these reports, the whole process of writing up can be greatly simplified by making a template report in Word. Into this template the details of each individual case can be inserted, either with macros or by using the Replace facility in Word. As the cases are nearly always identical in the nature of the injuries, the fine-tuning to individualise the report takes only a couple of minutes. Read through each report at the end to check for errors and remember to sign above your name and qualifications.

The most common reasons for solicitors returning reports are:

- Failure to answer specific questions.

- Failure to sign the report.

- Contradictory statements.

- Omission of details of injury chronology.

- Letter format (as opposed to report format).

As time goes on there are likely to be more and more solicitors firms requesting medico-legal work. The insurance industry foots the bill, passing on the cost to their policyholders. Sad though it is that the world is becoming increasingly litigious, GPs can, for once, benefit.

PRIVATE PATIENTS

Having private patients has always been possible as an NHS GP, and in some areas of the country a sizeable proportion of a practice's patients have traditionally paid for GPs normal services.

Remember that it is still not possible to charge registered NHS patients for core GP services, or those for which the practice is already being paid under additional or enhanced services. However, if there are enough patients willing to pay, then it may be profitable to offer them a completely private service.

What do private patients want? By paying for a private doctor, patients expect:

- A personalised service.

- To be able to see "their GP".

- To be exempt from rationing/public health issues.

- To have longer than the usual 10 minutes for their appointments.

- Telephone access, including from abroad.

- Appointments at convenient times, e.g. evenings and Saturday mornings.

- Pleasant surroundings.

- No crowded waiting room.

- To be able to discuss a range of subjects, including:
  - preventive/screening procedures;
  - services not generally available on the NHS, e.g. cosmetic surgery.

Tying all this in with NHS general practice is easily possible, especially if you are prepared to be flexible. Offering to speak to your private patients on the telephone when they ring for an appointment and to fit them in around normal surgery times will suit them nicely.

It looks professional if the patient is greeted by name by a pleasant receptionist. The invitation to go through to the "rooms" should be extended in person either by the doctor or the receptionist. Formality adds value, e.g. a handshake, door opening, standing to greet, etc. Take a thorough history at the first opportunity, especially including social, occupational, family and past medical histories. Computer use during the consultation should only be done with the patient's involvement, e.g. for downloading patient information leaflets.

Private patients may be prepared to pay to see you out-of-hours. This is entirely up to you, but should be agreed or otherwise at the earliest opportunity. It is quite reasonable to offer a bespoke private service during office hours only, with evenings/weekends by arrangement.

What should you charge? There are two main ways to calculate fees: either as an annual retainer or a fee-for-service. The latter is generally preferable as it discourages the abuse of the personal service.

Appointment lengths should be 30–45 minutes for an initial consultation and 15–20 minutes for a follow-up. Charging in units of 15 minutes is easiest, with rates anywhere from £30 to £100 per 15 minutes. Investigations, referrals and prescriptions should be charged as extra. Be prepared to waive your fee in particularly sensitive situations, e.g. deaths, especially for long-standing patients.

Patients usually expect to pay as they leave the surgery. Make sure you can accept cash, cheques and credit/debit cards. Install a swipe machine, for which you can expect to pay a rental equivalent to around 2% of the transactions. Avoid, where possible, having to send the patient an invoice. Chasing up overdue payments is time-consuming and embarrassing, and can result in lost fees.

In cities and large towns, some GPs can make a successful business entirely based on private GP services. If the numbers of private patients are insufficient, then other services, such as medico-legal or occupational work, can be tailored around the private patient service. For most GPs though, there will only be enough income by combining private and NHS work, and this is where some general principles are usefully operated.

GENERAL PRINCIPLES APPLYING TO EXTRA WORK

1. Extra work should be cost-effective

If you decide to build up a private practice, or to take on any extra work, there is an opportunity cost that must be priced. By doing the extra work, you may be unable to do something else, and that might run the risk of losing income. So long as the overall balance results in a net increase in profit, then the extra work is financially viable.

This applies particularly where the two competing types of work can only be done by you as a GP principal. If the work can be done by employing a doctor or nurse, then the only cost to your time is in the administration, and often even that can be delegated. It is not unusual, even in private practice, for employed doctors to see the patients, with the salaried doctor keeping, say, 30–50% of the fees generated.

2. Some extra work is more cost-effective than others

Doing four private vasectomies should generate enough income to cover the cost of a locum to cover the NHS surgery, leaving a decent profit margin. Taking the same time away from the surgery to do a clinical assistant session will barely cover the locum fees, and may even leave the practice at a net loss. Private work that can be dovetailed around existing services is particularly cost-effective, e.g. doing an insurance medical at the end of a surgery.

3. The principle of delegating work applies equally to NHS and private work

A secretary who can generate PMA reports frees up approximately 2 hours a week of a GP's time, saving the practice over £200 per GP per week in opportunity costs. Employing extra nursing time to undertake private contracts such as occupational health results in a good net profit for the practice. The amount of work that a practice can take on is potentially enormous, as long as partner involvement can be kept to a minimum.

4. Apply high standards

Employing a nurse of too low a grade for the job leaves the practice exposed to risk. Develop a tight specification, with room for safety. Similarly, taking on extra doctor work for which you are under-qualified can result in litigation. Good managerial input should ensure statutory requirements are met, e.g. health and safety. These should all be built into the costing before deciding whether to sign up to a new service.

PITFALLS

- Beware the ego trap – don't take on extra work for flattery or title. It is all too easy to believe that one is somehow a better person for agreeing to fill a vacant post, especially if there is the added status of a link with a specialist.

- Don't do it to escape from the grind. The thought of getting one or two sessions a week away from the routine surgery work can be appealing. Some doctors will do this even if the remuneration just covers the locum costs. Remember that new work is only novel for a finite time. Your paperwork will still be waiting for you when you get back to the practice.

- Don't incur the resentment of your partners. Losing money to the practice by taking on badly remunerated work should only be done with the full agreement of the other partners. Better still, take on work that earns your partners a visible profit.

- Avoid compressing existing surgery work into a shorter time. If you are to take on extra work, make sure you can delegate something else in return. Decide how busy you want to be – simply letting work mount up is not the way to maximise profit.

SETTING UP A PRIVATE SERVICE – THE VASECTOMY CLINIC

In general practice, as in any service industry, the earnings potential of the workforce is limited by their hours of availability. In order to earn the most, it becomes necessary to choose the work with the highest hourly rate of pay. If this work can be done without expensive overheads, then the profit margin increases the value of that work.

An example of this is providing a vasectomy service. With patients willing to pay upwards of £140 for the procedure, a half-hour's work is well rewarded. Fitted in at the end of a regular surgery, and performed in the practice's treatment room, the overheads are minimal. No locum is needed to cover absences from the practice, so long as the demand for the service is limited to one or two procedures a week. In some practices, this work generates more than twice the income from insurance and other reports combined.

The potential market for vasectomies is large. In big towns and cities there are plenty of men in the 25- to 50-year age range to provide enough patients for a private service to compete with the existing provision. In more rural or remote areas the advantages to patients of having the service on their doorstep are very attractive.

GPs can learn to do vasectomies by sitting in at a local clinic and being supervised as they operate. Ring the clinic and speak to one of the doctors, asking if they would mind if you watched a few vasectomies first. If they are worried about a local GP setting up in competition, it may be necessary to ask a clinic a little further afield.

Having been shown the essential steps of the procedure, it is a good idea to perform your first three or four vasectomies under the direct supervision of an experienced vasectomist. Minor surgical skills are possessed by most GPs, but the art of exposing the vas is probably the most important part of the operation to learn. Get a feel for the anatomy of each patient before starting the operation. Use plenty of local anaesthetic (10 ml lignocaine 2% with adrenaline). Get a 3-D image of the internal structures of the scrotum in your mind as you palpate the vas firmly between the thumb and index fingers of the left hand. Having made the skin incision, feel towards the vas with the tip of the fine Allis tissue forceps and make a wide grip, aiming to enclose the vas in the jaws of the forceps. Once this is successfully achieved on both sides, the rest of the operation is plain sailing.

Examples of consent forms, patient information leaflets and operating notes can be copied from Appendix 3. Semenalysis can be provided on a private basis from the local NHS laboratory and should cost about £5 per specimen.

The first few times you offer to provide a vasectomy service from your own surgery, it is a good idea to offer the patients the choice of either a referral to the established clinic or a free vasectomy in-house. It is essential to be honest about your level of experience. Many patients are happy to let their own GP do their vasectomy, especially if they have experienced other minor operations locally.

The equipment needed to perform a vasectomy is neither extensive nor expensive. The Central Sterilisation and Supplies Department of your local hospital should be able to supply operating packs for about £2 each. They should contain:

- Allis tissue forceps (three-toothed).

- Mosquito forceps (x2).

- Needle holder.

- Scissors.

- Fine, toothed forceps.

- Size 3 scalpel handle.

- Swab forceps.

In addition, each operation will need:

- Gauze swabs.

- Savlon.

- Plain vicryl or catgut suture (size 2/0).

- Number 11 scalpel blade.

- 10ml lignocaine 2% with adrenaline.

- 10ml syringe.

- Blue needle.

A simple adhesive dressing and two specimen jars with forms are also required.

An itemised summary of the costs of providing this service is given in Table 2.

	Cost (£)
Nurse	20
Semenalysis (x2)	10
Disposables	3
Sterilised equipment	2
Total	35
Fee per 30 minute operation	140
Profit per hour	210

Table 2. Costs for providing vasectomy service (per vasectomy)

Doing the occasional vasectomy is easy to fit in around existing surgery commitments. If the volume of work increases, there may be savings to be made on the overhead side, but taking a partner away from other clinical work will have an opportunity cost (such as lost GMS income) and may also involve locum expenditure. So it is important to gauge the workload to fit the available GP time, always maintaining an eye for overall profit. It is probably necessary to do no fewer than one or two vasectomies a month in order to maintain your skills.

Advertising

Once the vasectomy service has been established, advertising it to surrounding practices should increase the number of referrals. Most patients will come from neighbouring GPs, so it is to them that you should advertise. Highlight the value to patients of a local service, the competitive cost to the patient and the short waiting list.

Direct marketing to patients is fraught with risk, as the General Medical Council rules on advertising take a distinct dislike to patient canvassing. Furthermore, the GMC specifically forbids specialists from marketing directly to patients. It is not clear whether a GP providing a vasectomy service to patients of other practices is doing so as a GP or as a specialist, but there would be little difficulty making a case for disciplinary action if a patient complained.

It is reasonable to include the services of a GP in the practice leaflet, but only if those services are available to the patients of the practice. If services are available on a private, fee-paying basis they can also be included in the leaflet, but should be described as private services.

Advertising the service to the PCO should be done by the direct approach, and may result in a contract to provide patients in the area with the service. This would be in the form of a local enhanced service contract. Expect the fees to be lower than the private ones, but to offset this against the guarantee of a certain volume of work.

Working with other practices

One of the ways of increasing income by diversifying is to work collaboratively with other practices. There are several ways of doing this.

- Sharing staff.

- Seeing each others' patients.

- Mergers and take-overs.

- Co-operative work, e.g. out-of-hours.

- Buying in expertise.

Under the new GMS contract, and to some extent under PMS, the role of the practice manager is far more demanding than ever before. There is now a need for practice managers to take over the executive roles previously performed by partners, a need for vision and leadership, and a financial incentive to be efficient and thorough. As a result, practice managers are set to become more highly skilled, qualified and rewarded, and may therefore become too expensive for smaller practices. Only by sharing a practice manager will smaller practices be able to have the expertise they need to succeed financially.

This can be achieved by either employing a manager through one practice and co-opting them to the other practices, or by forming a joint employing body or locality group. This way of affording expert input does demand some degree of convergence of management structure between practices, but the able manager should have little difficulty accommodating different practices' systems.

The economy of scale theory goes right through the new GMS contract, with no weighting in the Carr–Hill formula to reflect the higher employment costs of small practices. Other staff can be shared to financial advantage as well as practice managers. Computer expertise, for example, can only be afforded by most practices on an ad hoc basis. With the emphasis in the new GMS contract on data handling, groups of practices can afford to employ dedicated computer expertise for both hardware and software problems, as well as data entry, searches and reporting.

Medical staff are an expensive commodity. Salaried GPs are now demanding salaries of £60,000 and so may be too expensive for a small practice that is just beginning to expand its services. Jointly employing a salaried doctor may free up enough time in a practice for one of the partners to do some outside work, with a net financial benefit to the practice.

MANAGER'S TIP

When employing salaried GPs make sure that there is no mismatch of expectations between the practice and the salaried GP. Set out clearly the tasks, duties and hours that the salaried GP will be expected to undertake.

The same applies to nursing staff. Spirometry, for example, is now required in all patients with chronic obstructive pulmonary disease. The equipment is not expensive, but there is an argument for having a dedicated member of the nursing team with the expertise to perform spirometry. This may not be affordable in every practice, but by contracting out the services of that nurse, both provider practices and user practices will benefit.

Alternatively, on the theme of spirometry, one practice could arrange for its patients to have their spirometry performed at a neighbouring practice. This would obviously need to be under a quality control contract and remunerated so as to benefit both practices. The same principle of shared facilities can be extended to other areas of the quality payments. For example:

- Access.

- Diabetes clinic.

- Smoking cessation adviser.

- Staff training.

Practices could cover each other to allow time for appraisal, revalidation, continuing professional development and practice management.

Some practices wishing to opt out of additional services may agree to subcontract them to a neighbouring practice, if the PCO payments for them were greater than the cost of paying the provider practice.

Out-of-hours may still be the best example of practices working co-operatively. After December 2004, the cost to the PCO of providing this service will rocket, and existing co-operatives will be in a strong position to bid for provision of the service, to the financial benefit of their members (see page 71).

Finally, GPs can provide a service to other practices by being employed as GP specialists.

GP SPECIALISTS

The new GMS contract makes the provision of some services a national requirement of every PCO. These services are too under-utilised in some areas to be required by every practice, so GP specialists will be involved in delivering a service to a number of practices. The PCO is the usual employer in this case. Other PCOs will have set up specialist services that can be provided by GPs within a locality. Examples include:

- Cardiology, e.g. echocardiography.

- Elderly care.

- Diabetes.

- Palliative medicine.

- Mental health, e.g. substance misuse.

- Dermatology.

- Musculoskeletal.

- Women and children.

- ENT.

- Homeless/asylum seekers.

- Procedures, e.g. vasectomy, endoscopy.

Training is usually provided for most of these activities and the remuneration is pitched at a level so as to make the roles appealing to well-paid partners.

As with any extra work, GPs should apply the rules to assess financial viability, as well as deciding where they would like their career to go.

- Beware the ego trap.

- Assess the opportunity costs.

- Don't desert your practice/partners.

- Delegate effectively.

SUMMARY – ACHIEVING A BALANCE

Diversity in general practice is a good thing; it adds interest, wealth and security. All GPs will do some non-GMS/PMS and some non-NHS work, and for some this will provide a sizeable portion of their profits. For most, however, their main NHS contract will provide the bulk of their earnings.

Choosing whether to take on extra work is a difficult decision. Not only is there a financial equation to consider, but this must be seen alongside the question of workload and lifestyle. How hard do you want to work?

As a rule of thumb, if you feel your workload is about right, then extra work must only be taken on by delegating tasks or buying in extra help. Only you can tell if your lifestyle as a GP is right for you at the moment.

The pursuit of wealth doesn't have to mean self-destruction and burnout. Intelligent and honest assessment should be applied to financial opportunities. Cherry-picking yields the best returns – leave the unripe fruit on the tree for someone else!

SKILL MIX

TRADITIONAL MODELS

Existing practice workforce structures have evolved to their present states out of necessity. Most practices have been owned by partners, who are usually all GPs, run by a practice manager, with support staff and practice nurses sharing the clinical and non-clinical work.

For a variety of reasons, some members of the team end up doing jobs that could be better done by someone else. For example, a GP sees a patient requesting a repeat prescription for an inhaler.

- First, the patient doesn't actually need to see a doctor just for this reason, but may not realise that.

- Secondly, the patient may not need to see anyone, if their repeat prescription is authorised and they have had an asthma check in the last year.

- As the patient has booked an appointment, the doctor decides to do the patient's asthma check anyway, believing this will help achieve the asthma target.

- After measuring the peak flow, giving smoking advice, recalculating the action plan thresholds and issuing the repeat prescription, the GP then feels out of time for ticking boxes on the computer.

- A Post-it sticker is left on the notes with "asthma check" written on it.

- The file clerk sees the sticker and thinks she had better put asthma check on the computer, and she knows there is a template for doing so.

- The box for annual asthma check is ticked.

When the list was generated for invitations to the asthma clinic, the patient's name didn't appear. Naturally the patient didn't attend, even though it was 11 months since their last check-up with the nurse. No record of smoking status got on to the computer, nor did advice to give up. These two targets were missed, and all because two members of the team thought they were helping to achieve them. Furthermore, the patient ignored the next year's invitation to see the nurse, believing that his GP did his asthma check-ups!

There are several reasons why these mistakes happened, and a variety of ways of helping to prevent them, but part of the problem lies in the traditional model of care.

- The patient who believes that GPs can do everything.

- The GP who thinks he can do everything.

- The file clerk who thinks she knows how to file everything.

- A computer that was only asked to tell half the story.

- The practice manager who has trusted people to do things properly.

Seeing patients is clearly a role for GPs and nurses, but, on the whole, GPs are better at diagnosing and treating illnesses, while nurses are better at monitoring chronic disease. Furthermore, nurses are generally better at sticking to protocol, and usually have longer appointment times than GPs.

The traditional notion that GPs, being generalists, can see and treat everything is outdated. General practice is far more complex than that. Not only do we need to develop watertight systems for effective teamwork; we need to include the patients in our evolving knowledge of the structure of a modern general practice.

The practice manager of the 1990s, who tried to put the GPs' ideas into practice, now has to change. Leadership is a quality that many managers have, but the importance that this quality contributes to the financial success of a practice cannot be overstated.

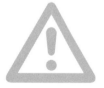

MANAGER'S TIP

Effective and efficient systems are the key to an effective organisation. Systems must be reviewed regularly with every member of the team, including GPs, to let them know how and when to play their part.

FINANCIAL PERSPECTIVE

When deciding on the skill mix requirements of your practice, there a number of rules to remember.

- The bottom line is profit.

- To make money you need to invest in staff.

- Staff will leave if they are undervalued.

- Teamwork is cheap.

- Under-utilised skills are costly.

- Have a 5-year plan.

There are two common pitfalls when planning skill mix investment: short-sightedness and tradition.

EXAMPLE

The Bleak Street Practice ran a tight ship under the old GMS contract, with staff costs well within budget and profits above Average Intended Net Remuneration. It seems to the partners that many of the new quality targets might be difficult to achieve without a disproportionate increase in workload both for themselves and the practice nurses. Their practice manager is worried about the effect of all this extra work on the morale of the nursing staff. After discussing the problem they decide to aim for a very modest quality target this year, and to see how things go. If they achieve their aims then the staff will feel rewarded and they could aim a little higher next year, possibly.

This approach to quality income is upside down. The practice is looking at the present structure and trying to please people, to maintain existing skill mix, and taking a year-by-year view.

Instead, they should look at the bottom line first – profit. What is the best way to achieve maximum profit for the practice from quality payments? Income can be maximised by achieving as many points as possible, and cash flow is optimised by aspiring to 1050 points in the first year.

How can the practice achieve 1050 points? This will come at a financial cost to the practice, but the rewards far outweigh the costs, so profits will rise. The essential elements are:

- A practice nurse can do the vast majority of the clinical work.

- Data management should be the responsibility of a dedicated and computer-literate person.

- Protected time is needed to set up, perform and monitor the quality system.

- Efficiency in the quality team will free up other members of staff.

The maximum amounts of money available in 2004/5 for reaching the top quality payments are:

Preparation payments per GP	£3000
1050 points at £25 each per GP	£26,250
Total, for the average three-partner practice	£87,750

Even if the practice needs to take on another full-time practice nurse to achieve the maximum quality score, there will still be plenty of room for profit.

Other members of staff involved in achieving the top score will include the practice manager, the data clerk and the GP with executive responsibility for quality. Their time is not cheap, but even factoring this into the costs will still leave the practice with a generous margin for their efforts. These non-patient roles also benefit from economy of scale, so the larger the practice the cheaper their time becomes. The average six-partner practice stands to gain a potential £30,000 a year profit per GP from hitting the top quality score.

Changing practice workforce structures

The advent of the practice-based contracts for GMS and PMS has changed the way medical manpower can be deployed. Instead of assuming that retiring partners or nurses need to be replaced with identikits, there are different ways of filling vacancies that are more lucrative. It is now the practice that decides how best to provide enough expertise to fill its contractual requirements.

The obvious examples are the salaried doctor and the nurse practitioner. The advantages are:

- Diversity adds colour.

- They take less out of the practice account than a profit-sharing partner.

- Numbers are no longer limited by a health authority staff budget.

- Recruitment is more straightforward.

- Future changes in manpower are more easily accommodated by 1- to 3-year contracts.

- Hours and roles are controlled by the practice.

The potential disadvantages are:

- Fringe benefits expected, e.g. medical indemnity costs.

- Reluctance to be flexible on hours.

- No guaranteed contribution to practice development/management.

- Commitment to paying salary even if profits fall.

Taking on extra employed staff in a climate of increasing opportunities and profitability is easy. It simply requires the vision to plan ahead and predict manpower needs. Overstretching the staff budget is fine, if increases in profitability can be demonstrated as the result.

Practices with a vacancy are in a good position to recruit a salaried replacement. Other situations where one might take on a salaried GP include:

- Expansion in number of registered patients.

- New financial opportunities.

- Predicted increase in profits.

- Desire to reduce partner workload.

Recruiting additional practice nurses is necessary when:

- Gearing up quality achievements.

- Taking on extra enhanced services.

- Securing private contracts for, say, occupational health.

- Employing nurses to subcontract to other practices/PCO.

Practice mergers are the ideal opportunity to reassess manpower needs. There are great economies of scale to be had under the new GMS contract. Taking on the list of a retiring single-handed GP will generate big rises in global sum, enhanced services and quality payments, with only one practice manager and a rationalised reception team still being needed. Employed staff can meet the extra clinical time required, including doctor hours, while the additional contributions to practice profitability will far outweigh their respective costs.

In the absence of such grand opportunities for change, one can still alter the skill mix of the other employed staff to the benefit of the practice. Remembering the rules of thumb above (page 54), consider that health care assistants can, among other things:

- Take blood.

- Do ECGs.

- Take blood pressures.

- Use a computer template.

- Perform spirometry.

- Measure peak flow.

Don't use your G-grade nurse for these tasks; she is too overqualified and expensive, compared to a health care assistant.

Separating out the skilled G-grade tasks from the simpler jobs will need the co-operation of the nursing team, a clear division of roles drawn up by the practice manager and a means of communicating these divisions to the patients via the reception staff. With new appointments, hours can be bought in as required. The employment of a health care assistant may, for example, free up enough G-grade nurse time to improve quality payments or to set up a triage system for urgent patient need.

Similarly, employing a highly qualified nurse practitioner might relieve the GPs of seeing enough urgent extras to enable them to meet access targets without a rise in workload. This will attract quality payments as well as enhanced service money, thus offsetting the nursing costs.

Planning for change in skill mix requires a fresh approach to practice structure. Look at the needs of the practice from a financial point of view, bearing in mind future opportunities and changes. Forget the current structure, lest it influences your free thinking. Don't think in terms of personalities so much as roles.

MANAGER'S TIP

To get the most out of skill mix, ask the question "Is someone doing something that a person on a lower grade/rate could legitimately and ethically do?", e.g. an E-grade nurse or even a health care assistant taking blood. Invest in a phlebotomist.

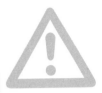

The adapting of existing staff should play on their individual strengths – for example, shifting from filing to data entry among those with an ability to be methodical, careful and computer-friendly.

A surplus of one type of worker can usually be dealt with by a combination of:

- Natural wastage.

- Training and encouragement to change.

- Disciplinary procedure.

- Practice expansion.

The future shape of general practice under the new GMS contract is going to be different from today. Being a partner is likely to be a coveted position, gained after several years' service as a salaried doctor. Practices will be bigger as the economies of scale are realised. Practice managers will be more highly skilled and rewarded. Nurses are going to play a greater role in the management of chronic disease and minor illness. Data management is to be the key to financial success, with a greater emphasis on staff computer training and skill.

This position can be reached more quickly by those practices with the courage to change. Sticking to the good old way of doing things will simply see the erosion of partners' pay packets.

EXAMPLE

The Bleak Street Practice in the example above tried a different approach. Their practice manager calculated the potential income from achieving the different quality standards and saw that there was a lot to be gained from going for the maximum score. The partners were convinced by this and decided to help find the best way of achieving the maximum number of points.

The members of the practice nurse team were all excited by the idea of aiming for the top score and were keen to do as much of the clinical work as possible, while recognising that more help would be needed doing their usual work. Similarly, the administrative staff thought it would be possible to fine-tune the recording of quality data by making the data clerk's time ring-fenced for the task.

The practice manager had a number of tasks to complete on her way to achieving all the organisational standards, and felt this could best be done by delegating some of her other work to the senior receptionist.

Having mapped out all the tasks needed to achieve the maximum quality target, it was clear that the practice needed to take on another half-time G-grade practice nurse and a half-time health care assistant, and to increase the data clerk's hours by five a week. The shift of chronic disease management to the nurses would free up enough GP time to enable advanced access to work, while providing spaces for the doctors to solve clinical problems thrown up by the chronic disease nurse appointments.

It was felt that these changes could start immediately but would take 2 years to achieve in full. The emphasis on maximising profits was consistent with the practice's 5-year business plan, and the aim of going for the top score in quality was a good motivator for the staff.

The partners charged their manager with the task of achieving their shared goal, and in return promised to comply with her request that they change the way they recorded certain data during consultations and allowed themselves to be subject to regular performance audits.

ACCOUNTANT'S TIP

Being a relatively large practice with a weighted list size of 10,376, this practice stands to earn £148,565 from quality points in 2004/5, rising to £237,705 the following year. Clearly, this is more than enough to cover the additional costs of achieving the maximum targets, leaving a healthy margin for practice profits.

SUMMARY

Never take skill mix for granted. The traditional model of general practice structure has served the profession well for almost 50 years, but its time is over. Under the new GMS and PMS contracts, the practice has complete freedom to decide the shape of its workforce. It can make a partner of any doctor, nurse, manager, spouse or even cleaner if it so chooses. It can employ as many doctors as it likes. It can get nurses to do all the work of generating income. It can opt in and out of services. It can mix private and NHS work.

Choosing the right staff for the job is an essential task in shaping the practice. Like moulding a lump of clay, it is infinitely pliable. With firm hands you can make your practice whatever you want it to be.

PRACTICE SIZE

INTRODUCTION

Under the Red Book, the average list size was a useful tool for analysing practice finances. Income tended to go up as list sizes rose. The average figure of about 1900 patients per full-time equivalent GP could be used to compare a practice's income with the national average. Once a figure of about 2000 patients per GP was reached, practices had to think about closing their lists, applying to take on additional partners to cope with rising demand, or losing income by taking on locums, assistants or retainers.

The situation now is very different. No longer will the appointment of a new partner attract additional funding in the form of a basic practice allowance. The GMS income a practice receives is based on:

- The patient list (global sum/MPIG).

- Practice performance (quality payments).

- Range of services (enhanced services).

These are all influenced by the number of patients belonging to the practice, with a linear increase in income with patient numbers. At face value, it therefore seems appropriate to advise practices to adopt as large a list size as possible in order to maximise income.

ECONOMY OF SCALE

The global sum payment does not take account of the relatively higher costs to small practices of employing staff. Every practice needs a manager, but whereas the large practice has a bigger income to contribute to that cost, the smaller practice must find the same cost from a smaller global sum. Again, the evidence points to the financial advantage of the larger practice.

The practice manager of today is working largely in a strategic/executive role. The administrative tasks of the practice can and should be delegated to senior reception staff or a deputy practice manager. This structuring increases costs but improves practice efficiency and financial success. It is only affordable by larger practices.

The strategic role of the modern practice manager is a commodity that must be available to every practice. For example, at least 160 of the quality points are for organisational work performed by the practice manager as a one-off act. The practice must achieve these or forfeit the income from them – a considerable sum. Completing the tasks required for these points will take as long for the practice manager of the small practice as it does for the manager of a large practice. Employing managers of the same ability costs the same irrespective of practice size.

The economy of scale suggests that larger practices are now at a considerable financial advantage, compared with their smaller counterparts.

Other staff

Economies of scale also apply to other employed staff to some extent. Achieving the highest possible quality score may only be achievable, even in small practices, by having staff whose dedicated role is data entry/extraction or seeing patients for the purpose of attaining quality targets. Admittedly, the more patients you have, the more times you need to enter data, but once a system is up and running, the workload does not increase linearly with patient numbers. A well-run diabetes clinic does not become twice as expensive to run by doubling the number of patients using it. Similarly, the costs of running the clinic do not halve if the patient demand is reduced by 50%.

Medical staff

All practices have a minimum requirement for a certain number of doctors to be available to see patients; not only to meet demand, but to meet access targets and appointment lengths, and to cover emergencies and extras. The number of doctors needed is dictated by the patient numbers, patient demand, practice skill mix and the appointment system.

Here, there is a linear relationship between patient numbers and medical staffing need, so the economy of scale appears not to apply. However, this basic need can be met as well by salaried medical staff as by the partners.

While a salaried doctor costs the practice about £65,000 a year, the average partner should expect to be costing the practice a lot more. So there is an advantage in employing salaried doctors as opposed to partners, at least from the point of view of overall practice profitability.

There is no financial disincentive for practices to do this. The money coming into the practice is the same irrespective of the status of the doctors.

DOWNSIDE OF THE LARGE PRACTICE

Is it more difficult for the large practice to achieve quality points? Experience does not support this notion. In comparative audits some practices are better organised than others, with achievement spanning a wide range, but there are as many large practices in the top quartile as there are small practices.

Large practices have no more difficulty achieving high standards than small practices. So long as the staff numbers are adequate for the task and the practice is managed as a unified team, there is no disadvantage in being big.

Where large practices often have difficulty is in getting all the partners to agree on a course of action. Generally, there are as many opinions about a subject as there are doctors to give an opinion. The bigger the partnership the more complex the decision-making. Herein lies another example of the value of the executive role of the practice manager – the ability to herd cats!

MANAGER'S TIP

Be prepared to take the lead and to suggest the unthinkable.

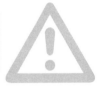

The other situation where the larger practice will lose out financially is where it opts out of additional services. Take out-of-hours (OOH), for example. The average GP with 1833 patients currently stands to lose £6000 a year from the global sum by opting out of OOH in December 2004. The effect of weighted practice list size is to increase this loss of income in proportion to patient numbers. To balance this, however, the cost of remaining as a purchaser of OOH services is also proportional to list size.

ACCOUNTANT'S TIP

Economies of scale in large practices will be diluted by opting out of anything.

PRACTICE VS PARTNERSHIP

Increasingly, under the GMS contract, and PMS also, there needs to develop a difference between the practice size and the partnership size. While decision-making is best performed by a small number of partners with an able practice manager, practice profitability is maximised by the practice with the larger number of patients.

This divergence is almost alien to many GPs, who have worked under a tightly regulated system of individual doctors' lists being directly tied to income.

Dentists have been aware of this beneficial arrangement for many years. Partnership is the final goal in a dentist's career, to be achieved, with luck, after several years' service as an associate. Other professionals such as architects, accountants and solicitors employ the same model. The thing they all have in common with the new GMS contract is that the income their practices receive is based on the total amount of work they do, not on the number of partners.

OPPORTUNITIES FOR CHANGE

If there is a desire to maximise profits:

- Practices should think big.

- State this in the business plan.

- Aim to increase the practice list size.

- Put a complete halt on taking on new partners.

- Employ enough staff to achieve the highest targets.

- Take on salaried doctors when the workload demands it.

Opportunities for change happen at practice level due to:

- The retirement of a partner.

- The desire of a partner to become salaried in exchange for income security and/or release from managerial duties.

- Local expansion in population.

- The closed list that can reopen.

- Partners increasing outside work.

- Change of practice manager or key members of staff.

Neighbouring practices may provide opportunities due to:

- Recruitment problems.

- Inadequate management.

- Failing targets.

- Opting out of additional services.

- Not taking on enhanced services.

- Closed lists.

- Single-hander retirement.

If none of the above opportunities seems likely in the near future, what are the options for practices wishing to grow?

Small practices can achieve the economy of scale by jointly employing expensive staff such as practice managers or dispensary managers. The member of staff would need to be employed by one of the practices under a written contract of shared hours with the neighbouring practice.

Groups of more than two practices could usefully join forces in order to take on rarely used expertise, such as specialist nursing or computer expertise.

Providing out-of-hours in a co-operative is a good example of the large group of practices working successfully, albeit for only one aspect of GPs' work.

Co-operation in achieving quality targets also pays off. For example, the practice with the successful, well-established diabetes clinic may be willing to see a neighbouring practice's patients if that practice can help to achieve, say, access targets.

Summary

Small practices were able to thrive under the Red Book because they were treated preferentially for staff funding, and a sizeable chunk of income related to partner numbers.

The new GMS contract provides no such advantage. There are, however, ways in which GPs in small practices can still maintain a decent profit by working in co-operation with their neighbours.

On the whole, though, there are great economies of scale in modern general practice that reward an expansionist policy. Practices with large lists, headed by small numbers of partners, are the best way to maximise profits. Partnership is likely to become the sought-after pinnacle of the aspiring GP's career, after several years as a salaried doctor in general practice.

OUT-OF-HOURS (OOH)

INTRODUCTION

The traditional role of the GP being available all hours has long been eroded out of necessity. The ever-increasing demand from patients to receive medical care outside normal hours has made it impossible for family doctors to deliver a service to their patients 24 hours a day, 365 days a year.

Under the old GMS contract, doctors were obliged to provide a service 24 hours a day and, for the sake of organisational cost-effectiveness, this was usually via an extended rota of either the partners of one or two practices, a co-operative of several local practices or by delegating to a deputising service.

The new GMS contract gives individual practices the choice of whether or not to provide out-of-hours (OOH) care. This choice can be expressed by April 2004 and exercised nationally by December 2004. After that time the responsibility for providing out-of-hours falls to the PCOs.

Out-of-hours is defined as 6.30 p.m. to 8.00 a.m. Monday to Friday, all weekend, Bank holidays and National holidays.

Choosing to opt out of out-of-hours (OOH) is a decision governed by several factors.

- The cost in terms of lost income.

- The profit in terms of income from working for the PCO doing OOH.

- The desire of the individuals to provide a more traditional OOH service.

- The opportunity to work after hours to boost other earnings.

Before looking at the financial implications, consider an average practice of three or more doctors. The chances are that there will be as many opinions on out-of-hours as there are doctors. In most practices there will be strong opinions on working unsocial hours, with the majority disliking the work but also dependent upon the income from it. First, it is important to come to a consensus on what the practice must say to the PCO. Remaining as a provider of out-of-hours after December 2004 would need the agreement of all members of the practice. It is not possible for some partners to opt out and others to continue as providers. The decision is practice based because the contract would be practice based.

That is not to say that a practice that opts in has committed all its partners to doing the work. It is perfectly reasonable for a practice to cover its patients out-of-hours by using less than the full number of partners to do the work. Large practices may find it more cost-effective to employ salaried staff to do some or all of the work out-of-hours.

Small practices in remote areas, while not having much choice but to continue providing cover, may be able to get by with one or two partners and locum help to continue providing a service.

Both systems allow for individual members of opted-in practices to personally opt out of doing the work. A corresponding adjustment to income would be needed in the practice accounts, by making out-of-hours payments a prior share.

HOW TO OPT OUT

If your practice decides to opt out of out-of-hours, make an early approach to the PCO stating as much. Put your request in writing, keeping a copy on file. State which aspects of the out-of-hours you may be prepared to cover, e.g. Saturday mornings, evenings until 11.00 p.m., early mornings. Make sure you state that these hours will only be covered as a local enhanced service provider, not on a voluntary basis. Offer to meet the PCO to discuss terms.

THE FINANCIAL IMPLICATIONS OF OPTING OUT

Until April 2004, all practices are obliged to continue providing out-of-hours care. During that time, the work is considered to be an additional service and the remuneration for doing so is reflected in the global sum/MPIG. From December 2004, all practices should have the opportunity to opt out, at which point the estimated average cost per GP will be £6000. This is based on 1800 patients with average weighting under the Carr–Hill formula. Therefore, the cost of opting out will be greater for practices with larger lists and above-average Carr–Hill weighting.

However, the true cost of opting out is less than this. While continuing to provide services under co-operative or deputising arrangements, most practices have to subsidise the NHS by paying to belong to an out-of-hours service themselves. By opting out, practices are effectively switching from being a service commissioner to a service provider, while the GPs of that practice have the option of continuing or relinquishing their work as providers.

So, the average £6000 can be reduced by the net amount GPs pay to belong to a co-operative or deputising service. The resulting loss of income then fails to incur income tax at 40%, thus reducing the net cost per GP. This is the true cost per GP of opting out of out-of-hours.

COST COMPARISON WITH OTHER INCOME STREAMS

The sum of £6000 can be earned by:

- Achieving 80 points on the quality scale.

- Completing 100 PMA reports.

- Doing 43 vasectomies.

- Writing 24 articles of 2000 words for the average GP newspaper.

- Working one session a week as a GP specialist.

- Managing 60 anticoagulated patients.

- Working one night a month for a commercial OOH service.

- Working one session as a GP/CPD Tutor.

MANAGER'S TIP

Undertaking another activity to replace the £6000 lost by opting out of out-of-hours can have other spin-offs for the practice by individuals developing skills and interests that are certainly not stimulated by OOH.

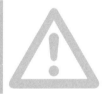

WORKING FOR THE PCO DOING OUT-OF-HOURS

PCOs need to commission out-of-hours care for large populations within the short time frame of 12 months, in a country with a GP recruitment crisis, in areas where the service is currently delivered to the great satisfaction of the vast majority of the patients.

Inevitably there will be an approach to the current providers of out-of-hours to continue to do so. The important thing for GPs is to value their services at market value, not on the charitable basis of the past. Co-operatives that employ GPs full-time to do out-of-hours are currently paying £85–100k for a 40-hour week. This works out at about £50 per hour, or £500 for an overnight shift.

If GPs can be persuaded to continue their out-of-hours co-operative arrangements, they could bid to provide the service themselves, at a commercial rate, and earn an additional £18–20k (minus the £6000 for the practice opt-out).

If this seems unlikely, the alternative is to offer to work for the PCO. This avoids the financial risk of running a co-operative, and should provide GPs with the opportunity to do the shifts they want, rather than having to take a turn at all shifts. The practice will still lose the £6000 for having opted out, but those GPs who want to boost their income are able to do so.

Don't forget that Saturday mornings are also out-of-hours under the GMS contract. PCOs will have great difficulty providing this service without the help of established GP services. Providing a Saturday morning emergency surgery could form the basis of a local enhanced service, but the contract price would have to be right. If a practice can earn more by seeing its quality target patients on a Saturday morning, then that may preclude the provision of a badly priced emergency surgery.

An example contract price is:

GP time	3 hours at £100 per hour	£300
Receptionist	3.5 hours at £15	£ 52.50
Overheads at 50%		£176.25
	Total	**£528.75 per week or £26,438 per year**

COMPETITION FOR GPs WANTING TO PROVIDE OUT-OF-HOURS

According to the NHS Confederation, out-of-hours services can be provided by a variety of means. The responsibility falls to the PCO to commission whichever system provides the most cost-effective cover. The options include, but are not confined to:

- GPs in Accident and Emergency departments.

- NHS Direct/NHS24.

- Paramedics.

- Walk-in centres.

- District nursing services.

- Minor injury units.

- Commercial deputising services.

- GP practices.

- GP co-operatives.

- PCO-employed OOH GPs.

There is no stipulation that a GP must be involved in the service, but the standards of the Out-Of-Hours Review must be met if the tender is to be awarded.

BIDDING TO PROVIDE OUT-OF-HOURS

Practices wishing to bid for the provision of OOH should look at the problem from the view of the PCO. How much would it cost to set up an alternative service? Are there already services in place that could be expanded to take on OOH care, such as NHS Direct? What would it cost to employ enough doctors to provide care for the whole PCO area out-of-hours? What would a deputising service charge?

With these answers it becomes easier to get a benchmark figure for a successful competitive tender. When approaching the PCO, stress the benefits of your proposal.

- Experience in providing out-of-hours care over many years.

- The value of local knowledge.

- A ready-made system for:

  – NHS communications
  – employment of staff
  – the provision of premises within the PCO area
  – familiarity with complaints
  – audit
  – appraisal.

Talk to other practices in your area. A joint approach to the PCO is likely to be more successful. Discuss the way forward with the rest of your co-operative and consider putting in an early bid to the PCO. Remember, you are very likely to be in the driving seat, especially in the early days of the new GMS contract. OOH will be entirely voluntary, so don't reduce the price just for the sake of appearing reasonable. Practices in remote parts of the UK should be able to negotiate very lucrative terms for OOH as an enhanced service.

Pricing out-of-hours

Most GP co-operatives already run as limited companies, with accounts going back over several years. These can be used as the basis of a pricing mechanism for a bid. Remember to allow for the loss of the OOH development fund money, and to increase the doctors' payments in line with commercial rates.

If the PCO are going to commission OOH from your co-operative, they will want it to provide cover for all the practices in the area, to relieve them of their responsibility. If there is a mixture of deputising and co-operative cover in the area at present, remember to include the extra coverage in your pricing and manpower calculations.

If you are bidding as an individual practice, you will need to take account of neighbouring bids, co-operative bids and commercial deputising service bids. If you think the competition is too strong, then make an approach to join forces.

Co-operatives as providers of out-of-hours after December 2004

Co-operatives should ensure that their GP members are willing to undertake out-of-hours work after December 2004 for an enhanced rate. It will be necessary to sign members up to a certain number of shifts per month, but this should be made voluntary, variable and flexible to encourage participation. By employing full-time doctors as well, the co-operative should be able to guarantee that all hours are covered. Produce rotas at least 3 months in advance and have a second on-call system for unexpected absences.

The existing infrastructure and employment patterns for drivers, receptionists and call handlers should be able to continue, and should be increased to allow for any additional practices that will need to be covered.

Employing doctors on full-time OOH contracts is not a new venture for some co-operatives. So long as the pricing is adequate, there should be little problem recruiting doctors with at least the Joint Certificate level of experience. Salaries of between £85,000 and £100,000 for a 40-hour week have been advertised in the last 2 years. It would not be unreasonable to expect the full-time doctors to cover the nights, with a rota of local GPs covering the evenings, for the same rate of pay.

Executive members of the co-operative board should be well remunerated for running the service. In fact, the ideology of co-operative working will be changed by the commercialisation of the doctors' pay rates. In return for receiving a commercial rate, participating doctors should not expect to share in the profits of the company, if there are any. Directors' salaries can be built in to the pricing of the contract.

Of course, it may be better to offer participating doctors a share of the profits in addition to a good salary. This will help recruitment, generate good will and encourage participation in complete rota coverage. Directors who work a share of the shifts demonstrate the fairness of their salaries compared to their non-director participating colleagues.

SUMMARY

Out-of-hours is the biggest change to affect GPs under the new GMS contract. Not only have the new arrangements allowed GPs to significantly limit their workload; they have recognised the high value attached to a service that was previously provided to the NHS on the cheap.

GPs planning to earn big incomes have a variety of ways of using the new OOH arrangements to their advantage. Simply by ensuring they can continue to work the same number of hours as they did previously, GPs should see this aspect of their remuneration triple or even quadruple.

ACCOUNTANT'S TIP

Large group practices, especially those with above-average list sizes, stand to lose the most from opting out of out-of-hours. For them it may be best to delay opting out until 2005/6, when the loss will be better cushioned by the big increase in quality payments from £75 to £120 per point.

By being proactive, talking to the PCO and mobilising local GP support, practices should be able to put themselves in a strong position for future financial success.

QUALITY

INTRODUCTION

A considerable proportion of a GP's GMS income can come from quality payments. Furthermore, unlike the global sum, the amount of money available to a practice for quality can be increased by careful means. It is essential, therefore, to do everything possible to maximise this source of income; not only is it good for the finances; it is good medicine. There is no reason why the practice should be unable to achieve the maximum payment available under the quality payment scheme. Much of the work can be delegated to well-organised staff and, even though this has cost implications, the benefits to the profits are well worth it.

In essence, the clinical quality payments are earned by reaching target levels of achievement in the management of the 10 chronic diseases:

- Coronary heart disease and left ventricular dysfunction.

- Stroke/transient ischaemic attacks.

- Hypertension.

- Diabetes.

- Chronic obstructive pulmonary disease.

- Epilepsy.

- Hypothyroidism.

- Cancer.

- Mental health.

- Asthma.

Organisational quality payments are earned by achieving set standards for:

- Records and information about patients.

- Patient communication.

- Education and training.

- Practice management.

- Medicines management.

- Length of consultations.

- Patient surveys.

- Access.

Additional services also attract quality points by achieving set standards for:

- Cervical screening.

- Child health surveillance.

- Maternity services.

- Contraceptive services.

THE KEY TO SUCCESS

Achieving the maximum income available to your practice under the quality payment scheme is easily possible. The key is to make top quality achievement a number one priority, by:

- Investing in the right staff to do the work.

- Monitoring progress constantly.

- Sharing your aims with the whole practice team.

- Including the goal in your business plan.

- Attention to detail.

- Intelligent manipulation of the system.

Practice nurses can do the bulk of the work of seeing the patients. Nurse practitioners are not essential. In fact, an F-grade practice nurse can carry out all the clinical work involved in achieving the quality targets. This assumes you have a system for training nursing staff in-house and a reliable mechanism for nurse-to-GP referral. Adequate investment in nursing time is paramount. The cost of this is returned to the practice many times over in increased quality payments.

The other essential staff are:

- A partner to oversee the clinical standards.

- A good practice manager to establish systems and manage audits.

- A dedicated computer clerk.

- A well-organised and meticulous clinic co-ordinator.

MANAGER'S TIP

Much of the GMS contract is about collating, recording and retrieving data. This is not a difficult job but it requires absolute attention to detail. It is best done by a designated clerk who takes a pride in routine work. Requiring your data clerk to multi-task may not be best. The last thing you want to happen is that this role becomes neglected because cover is needed for a sick receptionist.

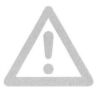

METHOD OF PAYMENT

Money earned under the quality umbrella is paid to practices in three ways:

1. **Preparation payments.** These are available to practices to help start the process of data collection. They are small (£9000 on average per three-doctor practice in 2003/4, £3250 in 2004/5 and nothing thereafter) and are calculated from the allocation formula.

2. **Aspiration payments.** These are paid in advance to practices, in anticipation of reaching a presumed level of quality. At the time of writing, they are equal to one third of the target quality payment. For cash flow purposes it is better to try to maximise the aspiration payments by declaring a high target. There is no penalty for failing to achieve a target.

3. **Achievement payments.** These are based on the total number of points scored by the end of the financial year, and are paid minus the aspiration payments already received for that year. The maximum achievable is 1050 points (worth £75 per 5500 patients on average in 2004/5, rising to £120 for 2005/6, or £126,000 for the average three-doctor practice).

ACCOUNTANT'S TIP

Given that there is £1.3 billion available for quality in 2004/5, this assumes that the average practice will achieve just over 50% of the points.

The rise in quality payments from £75 to £120 in 2005/6 is huge, particularly for practices with a larger weighted list size. For example, the practice with a weighted list size of 14,217 achieving 850 quality points will see its quality payments rise from £164,788 in 2004/5 to £263,661 the following year – an increase of nearly £100,000 for no extra work.

Before looking at the specific details of how to achieve the targets for the individual areas, there are some general points applicable to them all.

- Maximising income does not come simply from providing high-quality medical management. The keys to success are good data handling, ruthless tracking of patients and minimising overheads.

- It is important to distinguish between data that contribute towards a target payment (e.g. smoking status in hypertensives) and data that do not (e.g. annual U&Es in hypertensives).

- Computers are the hub of a practice's clinical quality payment scheme. Without all clinicians using the computer adequately there is no chance of achieving maximum payments. At the time of writing, there are still 168 practices in the UK that do not use a computer system at all!

- Templates are the key to successful computer use (see page 11).

- Patients who fail to turn up when invited for chronic disease monitoring should be recorded correctly on the computer as having DNAd (see Exclusions, below).

- Patients who do turn up should have the full range of parameters measured and recorded on the computer. Partial recording loses money.

- Nurses are cheaper than doctors. Employing a nurse to undertake chronic disease monitoring is more cost-effective than getting the partners or a salaried doctor to do it.

- Between them, the partners should retain ownership of all the chronic diseases that attract quality payments. An ethos of "the buck stops here" is an invaluable tool in ensuring maximum payments are achieved.

COMPUTER TEMPLATES

Setting up a high-quality, template-based system for computer recording of data has been explored in the chapter on The Ideal Practice, and in Appendix 1.

EXCLUSIONS (EXCEPTION REPORTING)

Recording patients who fail to turn up for chronic disease monitoring is essential. Those who do not attend after three written invitations can be removed from the denominator when calculating the proportion of patients achieving target. Patients who refuse screening can be removed after the first invitation, so long as the refusal is documented.

Furthermore, it is possible to exclude from the denominator patients who have recently joined the practice, or who have recently been diagnosed with the condition (in the last 9 months).

Other exclusions include patients for whom treatment is inappropriate, e.g. allergic/intolerant of a drug or terminally ill.

Patients on maximal treatment who still don't achieve the target should also be removed from the denominator.

The Read codes to use are:

8HA5 – "Follow-up refused"
9OX5 – "Influenza vaccine declined"
9N4I – "DNA diabetic clinic"
9N4J – "DNA cardiac clinic"
9N4L – "DNA hypertension clinic"

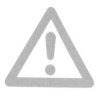

MANAGER'S TIP

The practice should have a written policy and protocol to pick up and record DNAs on the computer. This is particularly important when monitoring chronic diseases or even flu vaccination. At the end of the year, run a search on those patients on the disease register who have monitoring data missing and no record of exclusion. Look closely at their record. Enter a code for exclusion if it is clear they fit into one of the above groups.

GHOST PATIENTS

With any age–sex disease register, one of the biggest bugbears is the group of patients who don't actually have the disease. Run a computer search looking at the patients with a diagnosis of, say, angina and the date of their last blood pressure check. It's amazing to think that some of them haven't had a BP reading taken in the last 5 or 10 years! Now look closely at their individual records. Although they have an entry of angina some time in the past, there are several reasons why the patients may not actually have the condition. For example, angina may have been suspected but never confirmed, or even excluded after exercise testing. Ten years ago, the importance of recording accurately on the computer was not fully appreciated by clinicians and it was all too easy to enter "Angina" in the diagnosis section, with "suspected" or "possible" in free text.

These patients must be removed from the register if they don't have the condition. The correct way to record the above example would be to put "Chest pain" as the diagnosis and "angina suspected" in free text. Print off a list of each partners patients currently on the register and ask each to confirm, from memory, which patients have the condition. If there is any doubt, they should check the patient record. All patients without the condition must have all references to the bogus diagnosis removed from searchable areas of their computer record. Run the search again to confirm that those patients no longer appear. Culling these "ghost patients" from the disease register is the easiest way to improve your targets – and doesn't involve seeing a single patient!

MULTIPLE PATHOLOGY

When setting up call/recall systems for the monitoring of chronic disease, be aware of the fact that a considerable number of patients will be on more than one disease register. For example, a number of diabetes patients will also have hypertension or coronary heart disease.

It is wasteful and inefficient to invite those patients for annual review separately for each condition. Much of the lifestyle advice and many of the examinations and investigations overlap from one disease area to another, such as smoking and cholesterol. It is good medicine to consider a patient and all their diseases as a whole, and it makes financial sense to record all pertinent data at one opportunity. Cross-covering multiple disease areas will also help towards achieving points for the holistic care payments.

For example, many practices already run a diabetes clinic, with at least an annual review of all Type 2 diabetes patients. Those patients are having a blood test prior to their clinic appointment and being seen by a nurse and/or doctor with the results. If the patient also has hypertension, ischaemic heart disease or heart failure, then only one or two extra parameters will need to be recorded to complete the annual review of those conditions also.

A convenient computer link between disease templates can be set up to allow easy recording across the full range of disease areas for each patient (see Appendix 1).

ESTABLISHING A STRUCTURED ANNUAL REVIEW

For diseases such as coronary heart disease and diabetes, there are a lot of points and considerable financial reward available for achieving tight control and prescribing set drugs. The implication from this is that these patients will need to be seen annually by either a doctor or a highly qualified nurse who is able to change medication according to clinical criteria. In addition, there are many data areas that need to be covered that don't require a doctor, such as smoking advice.

Many of these data can be covered by writing to the patient in advance of their annual check-up, asking them to complete a questionnaire, which they then return to the practice. Depending on the disease, this can cover: smoking status, smoking advice offered, drugs taken (important for aspirin, which may be an OTC item), receipt of flu jab last winter and date of last seizure.

The invitation letter can also include instructions to attend for a blood test at least 2 weeks prior to the check-up, so that results are available when the patient is seen by the doctor/nurse. Patients should be given the opportunity to refuse an appointment at this stage and they can be excluded from the denominator (see above).

A member of staff should be responsible for keeping tabs on who has been invited and whether they turn up. Three invitations resulting in a DNA will result in the exclusion of patients from the denominator.

When the patients return their questionnaires, a member of staff, using the structured disease data grids described in the chapter on The Ideal Practice, should enter the data.

MONITOR YOUR PROGRESS

The achievement targets are measured for payment purposes at the end of each financial year. Don't wait until then to see how you're doing with your progress towards your target. Get into the habit of running searches on all clinical quality areas every month. That gives you plenty of time to address any projected shortfalls in performance.

INDIVIDUAL CLINICAL AREAS

The targets for achieving maximum payment are described under each disease heading, with an explanation of how best they can be achieved.

There are 10 categories of clinical quality indicator and a total of 76 indicators. Indicators are of two types. The first indicator in each category is whether or not the practice maintains a register of patients appropriate to the category and requires a Yes/No answer. A Yes answer is required for any further points to be earned in that category. The other indicator type is a percentage achievement for the indicator. To earn any points for an indicator the achievement must exceed 25%. The maximum achievement for which points can be earned is described in the text. Note that exceeding the maximum for an indicator will not earn any extra points.

SECONDARY PREVENTION IN CORONARY HEART DISEASE

CHD 1. The practice can produce a register of patients with coronary heart disease – 6 points.

Simply run a search of all registered patients with any record of a Read code starting with G3 (or G4 for Read 4 byte) for Ischaemic heart disease. Remember to make this a hierarchical search, i.e. to include patients with all codes beginning with G3, not just those having the G3 code in isolation. The elimination of ghost patients is crucial (see above). The prevalence should be around 3–5%, but should be compared with your PCO average. If there is a wide discrepancy, consider running a MIQUEST cardiovascular disease register query set.

CHD 2. Ninety percent of patients with newly diagnosed angina (diagnosed after 1 April 2003) are referred for exercise testing and/or specialist assessment – 7 points.

Clearly, the onus is on the doctors in the practice to refer new cases. As patients will not appear on the disease register until their first G3 code is entered on their computerised medical record, a prompt can be set up. Use the CHD register as the trigger for a guideline. Customise the guideline to include a prompt for referral. This will ensure that the referral prompt only appears the first time the patient is put on the register and not every time angina is entered.

If patients are diagnosed in hospital, make sure there is a computer entry for specialist assessment (e.g. 8H44 "Cardiology referral") put in their record upon receipt of the hospital letter. Exercise testing = Read code 3213.

CHD 3. Ninety percent of patients with coronary heart disease have a record of smoking status in the past 15 months, except those recorded as non-smokers – 7 points.

Inviting all CHD patients for a check-up once a year will cover this. The question of smoking status can be asked in the questionnaire enclosed with the invitation. Read codes are:

Non-smoker	137L
Never smoked	1371
Smoker	137R

CHD 4. Ninety percent of smokers in the CHD group have been offered smoking advice in the last 15 months – 4 points.

Smoking advice can be offered in the written invitation sent to all patients. For those attending their annual review, smoking advice can be offered if they smoke, and recorded (e.g. Read code 8CAL). Remember to exclude DNAs.

CHD 5. Ninety percent of CHD patients should have had a blood pressure reading recorded in the last 15 months – 7 points.

Again, at the annual review, the blood pressure can be taken and recorded on the computer. Read code = 246.

CHD 6. The last blood pressure reading should be less than 150/90 in 70% of CHD patients within the last 15 months – 19 points.

This is where the person seeing the patient needs to be able to alter the medication if necessary. If there are a lot of hypertensive CHD patients being seen, it makes sense that a doctor runs the clinic. Once good control is achieved in most people, then a nurse could run the clinic, referring to a doctor those patients above 150/90. Whoever takes the blood pressure should have responsibility for making sure the patient is not left for another year without further attempts to get a normal blood pressure reading onto the computer. Altering the medication, seeing the patient for follow-up, aiming for <150/90 and recording results are all essential. Remember those patients who can be excluded (see page 79).

CHD 7. Ninety percent of CHD patients should have had a total cholesterol measurement recorded in the last 15 months – 7 points.

When patients are invited for their annual check-up they can be asked to attend 2 weeks beforehand to have a blood test for total cholesterol. When the results come from the lab there must be a system in place for getting them onto the computer. This is best achieved by lab links. In the absence of links, the practice should have a policy of all cholesterol results being put onto the computer by a member of staff. Read code = 44P.

CHD 8. The latest total cholesterol result should be 5 mmol/l or less in 60% of CHD patients within the last 15 months – 16 points.

There is no upper age limit in the new contract for this parameter. Excluding patients above any age threshold will need to be negotiated. Until then the same applies as to blood pressure control. Titrating statin doses upwards can be done by a well-trained nurse, but the onus is on the person managing the condition to follow the patient up until they have either achieved target or reached the maximum tolerated dose. Either way, a computer entry needs to be made confirming successful completion for payment purposes.

CHD 9. Ninety percent of CHD patients are taking an antiplatelet/anticoagulant – 7 points.

This information will come from either the patient questionnaire or the repeat prescribing screen and must be checked at the annual check-up. There must be an entry less than 15 months old of either: a repeat prescription, salicylate prophylaxis (Read code 8B63) or aspirin allergy/intolerance. This will need updating at each annual check-up. Patients not fulfilling any of these will need to be started on aspirin or a suitable alternative (warfarin, clopidogrel, dipyridamole). The numbers are likely to be so small that an untrained nurse could refer all these cases to one of the doctors. Other useful Read codes are:

OTC aspirin	8B3T
Medication stopped, interaction	8BI6
Aspirin prophylaxis contraindicated	8I24

Warfarin contraindicated	8I25
Adverse reaction to warfarin	TJ421
Adverse reaction to salicylates	TJ53
History of aspirin allergy	ZV148

CHD 10. Fifty percent of CHD patients should be on a beta-blocker unless contraindicated – 7 points.

Contraindications include side-effects, but this must be recorded (Read code 8I26 "Beta-blocker contraindicated" or 8I36 "Beta-blocker refused"). Patients with stable angina and no history of myocardial infarction (MI) could question their need to start this therapy. The 8I26 code should get around this problem.

CHD 11. Seventy percent of MI patients diagnosed after 1 April 2003 should be on an angiotensin-converting enzyme (ACE) inhibitor – 7 points.

Most patients are diagnosed in hospital nowadays and are discharged on an ACE inhibitor. Make sure their repeat medication list includes this at their annual review. Read code 8I28 "ACE inhibitor contraindicated" should be used if there is any reason why the patient is not able to take an ACE inhibitor. Starting the patient on therapy should be by referral to one of the GPs. The Read code for myocardial infarction is G30.

CHD 12. The uptake of flu vaccine should be 85% in CHD patients – 7 points.

This can only be given between 1 September and 31 March. Patients attending for their annual CHD check between these dates should be immunised during their check-up. Unimmunised patients seen outside this range can only be advised to have the jab next time. However, patients can be excluded from this target if they have refused or failed to attend after three invitations to do so. Sending two reminders to CHD patients during the flu jab season is therefore important. Read codes to use are: 65E "Flu vaccination given" and 8I2F "Flu vaccination contraindicated".

MANAGER'S TIP

As with all chronic disease, make sure that you have a mechanism for recording and retrieving the fact that you sent an invitation and its subsequent refusal.

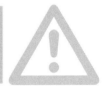

LEFT VENTRICULAR DYSFUNCTION

LVD 1. The practice can produce a register of patients with coronary heart disease and left ventricular dysfunction – 4 points.

In the G3 (CHD) group, search for G58 to include all heart failure patients, or G581 if you think you have been correctly coding for left ventricular failure. The incidence will be about 1% for patients under 75 and 8% for patients over 75, but it is worth checking with the PCO what they expect. Remove ghosts if you are too high. The numbers are small enough to warrant a closer look at individual patient records to confirm the diagnosis.

LVD 2. Ninety percent of patients with CHD diagnosed with left ventricular dysfunction after 1 April 2003 should have had an echocardiogram – 6 points.

The onus is on the doctors suspecting LVF to refer all patients for echo (now available by open access in many areas). It is important not to put a heart failure code on the computer until after the echo has confirmed the condition. This way the target should be 100%! Read code = 58531 "Echo abnormal".

LVD 3. Seventy percent of patients with CHD and LVF should be on an ACE inhibitor or A_2 antagonist – 10 points.

Existing patients may not be, but can be started on treatment by referral to a GP following their annual check-up. The disease template for LVF should have a box with the 8B6B Read code for ACE inhibitor prophylaxis, or 8I28 if ACE inhibitors are contraindicated (e.g. by being poorly tolerated).

Reward for CHD

A total of 121 points is available for reaching these targets. For 2004/5 this is worth an average of £8250 per 5000 patients, rising to £13,200 per 5000 patients from 2005/6.

STROKE AND TRANSIENT ISCHAEMIC ATTACK

STROKE 1. The practice can produce a register of patients with stroke and transient ischaemic attack (TIA) – 4 points.

Simply run a search of all registered patients with any record of a Read code starting with G61 for "Haemorrhagic stroke" and G64 for "Non-haemorrhagic stroke". Remember to make this a hierarchical search, i.e. to include patients with all codes beginning with G6, not just those having the G6 code in isolation. The elimination of ghost patients is crucial (see above). The prevalence should be around 0.2–0.3%, but should be compared with your PCO average. TIA=G65

STROKE 2. Eighty percent of strokes diagnosed after 1 April 2003 should have been confirmed by CT/MRI scan – 2 points.

It is therefore important not to enter a G6 code until the scan confirms the diagnosis. This is a message for the doctors who are likely to be seeing patients with suspected strokes, especially on home visits. A better Read code to use initially will be the one that reflects the symptoms/signs, e.g. F22 "Hemiplegia" or 1B65.11 "O/E collapse".

Letters from hospital confirming a stroke should have the Read code 5674 "CT scan" or 5693 "MRI abnormal" entered at the same time as the G6 code.

STROKE 3. Ninety percent of patients with TIA or stroke have a record of smoking status in the last 15 months except for recorded non-smokers – 3 points.

Write to all stroke/TIA patients once a year, inviting them for a check-up. Housebound patients may see the district nurse. Enclose a questionnaire asking about smoking status. Enter the replies on the computer. Exclude non-responders after three attempts. For Read codes see CHD section.

STROKE 4. Seventy percent of stroke/TIA patients who smoke should have been offered smoking cessation advice in the last 15 months – 2 points.

Strictly speaking, this advice does not have to be given, only offered. A face-to-face consultation is not specified. The questionnaire could include the question: "If you are a smoker, would you like to receive advice on how to give up?"

STROKE 5. Ninety percent of stroke/TIA patients should have had blood pressure recorded in the last 15 months – 2 points.

An annual invitation to all G6 patients should include the opportunity to have a blood pressure check. Patients unable to come to the surgery should be offered a visit by the district nurse. Refusers and non-responders after three letters should be excluded.

STROKE 6. The last blood pressure reading should be less than 150/90 in 70% of stroke/TIA patients within the last 15 months – 5 points.

Good liaison between the district nurse and GP are essential in achieving this. Altering medication to achieve target blood pressure can mean a series of house calls. Whoever takes the blood pressure should have responsibility for making sure the patient is not left for another year without further attempts to get a normal blood pressure reading onto the computer. Altering the medication, seeing the patient for follow-up, aiming for <150/90 and recording results are all essential. Remember those patients who can be excluded (see page 79).

STROKE 7. Ninety percent of stroke/TIA patients should have had a total cholesterol reading recorded in the last 15 months – 2 points.

At the same time as writing to the patient to invite them to come in for a check-up, a request can be made for them to have a blood test for total cholesterol. Those patients unable to come in can have their blood taken via the district nursing service. Nursing home staff can arrange blood testing on appropriate patients. All patients considered too frail/elderly should be excluded (see page 79).

STROKE 8. The latest total cholesterol result should be 5 mmol/l or less in 60% of stroke/TIA patients within the last 15 months – 5 points.

There is no upper age limit in the new contract for this parameter. Excluding patients above any age threshold will need to be negotiated. Until then the same applies as for blood pressure control. Titrating statin doses upwards can be done by a well-trained nurse or by liaison between the district nurse and the GP. The onus is on the person managing the condition to follow the patient up until they have either achieved target or reached the maximum tolerated dose. Either way, a computer entry needs to be made confirming successful completion for payment purposes.

STROKE 9. Ninety percent of patients with TIA or non-haemorrhagic stroke should be taking an antiplatelet or anticoagulant drug – 4 points.

This information will come from either the patient questionnaire or the repeat prescribing screen and must be checked at the annual check-up. There must be an entry less than 15 months old of either a repeat prescription, salicylate prophylaxis (Read code 8B63) or aspirin allergy/intolerance. This will need updating at each annual check-up. Patients not fulfilling any of these will need to be started on aspirin or a suitable alternative (warfarin, clopidogrel, dipyridamole). The numbers are likely to be so small that an untrained nurse could refer all these cases to one of the doctors. See CHD section for other Read codes.

STROKE 10. The uptake of flu vaccine should be 85% in stroke/TIA patients – 2 points.

This can only be done between 1 September and 31 March. Patients having their annual check between these dates should be immunised during their check-up. Unimmunised patients seen outside this range can only be advised to have the jab next time. However, patients can be excluded from this target if they have refused or failed to attend after three invitations to do so. Sending two reminders to stroke/TIA patients during the flu jab season is therefore important.

Reward for stroke/TIA

A total of 31 points is available for reaching these targets. For 2004/5 this is worth an average of £2114 per 5000 patients, rising to £3382 per 5000 patients from 2005/6.

HYPERTENSION

BP 1. The practice can produce a register of patients with hypertension – 9 points.

Simply run a search of all registered patients with any record of a Read code starting with G2 (or G3 for Read 4 byte) for Hypertension. Remember to make this a hierarchical search, i.e. to include patients with all codes beginning with G2, not just those having the G2 code in isolation. The elimination of ghost patients is crucial (see above). The prevalence should be around 6–10%, but should be compared with your PCO average.

BP 2. Ninety percent of patients with hypertension should have at least one record of smoking status – 10 points.

This can be asked at the 6-monthly blood pressure check and entered on the computer. A line for smoking status will be needed on the hypertension data grid.

BP 3. Ninety percent of hypertensive smokers should have been offered smoking cessation advice – 10 points.

If there is a prompt on the computer record, e.g. a line in the data grid, to be filled in then this advice can easily be remembered. Although only one record is ever required for hypertension, a significant number of patients have co-morbidity. Those with diabetes, CHD, stoke/TIA, asthma and COPD will require an entry for smoking advice at least every 15 months. Get into the habit of ticking the box at every opportunity.

BP 4. Ninety percent of patients with a history of hypertension should have had a blood pressure reading taken in the last 9 months – 20 points.

Hence the need for 6-monthly checks as standard. Set repeat prescribing intervals at 6 months. Use overdue repeats as prompts for invitations for a check-up. Patients not on medication should be screened to exclude ghosts (see page 80). Those on lifestyle advice only should be invited to re-attend every 6 months. Failure to comply with three written requests results in an exclusion from the denominator (see page 79).

BP 5. The last blood pressure reading should be less than 150/90 in 70% of hypertension patients within the last 9 months – 56 points.

This is where the person seeing the patient needs to be able to alter the medication if necessary. A nurse could be seeing the patients, referring to a doctor those patients above 150/90 or asking for advice from a doctor at the time of the nurse consultation. Whoever takes the blood pressure should have responsibility for making sure the patient is not left for another 6 months without further attempts to get a normal blood pressure reading onto the computer. Altering the medication, seeing the patient for follow-up, aiming for <150/90 and recording results are all essential. Remember those patients who can be excluded (see page 79).

Reward for hypertension

A total of 105 points is available for reaching these targets. For 2004/5 this is worth an average of £7159 per 5000 patients, rising to £11,455 per 5000 patients from 2005/6.

DIABETES

As a general principle, there are two sources of data on diabetics: hospital outpatient letters and in-house data from the practice's diabetes clinic. The former are valuable pieces of paper and should not be filed until their data have been extracted by a member of staff who knows what to look for.

DM 1. The practice can produce a register of patients with diabetes – 6 points.

Simply run a search of all registered patients with any record of a Read code starting with C10 (or C2 for Read 4 byte) for Diabetes mellitus. Remember to make this a hierarchical search, i.e. to include patients with all codes beginning with C10, not just those having the C10 code in isolation. The elimination of ghost patients is crucial (see page 80). The prevalence should be around 2.5%, but should be compared with your PCO average. The incidence is set to double over the next 10 years.

DM 2. Ninety percent of patients with diabetes should have a record of Body Mass Index (BMI) in the last 15 months – 3 points.

The interval between clinic attendances should be no more than 1 year. Weight measurement should be an integral part of the clinic work-up, with height being recorded at least once (e.g. new patients). Most computer systems convert weight to BMI, but if not, use BMI = kg/m^2. Preferred Read code = 22K.

DM 3. Ninety percent of patients with diabetes should have a record of smoking status in the past 15 months, except those recorded as non-smokers – 3 points.

Inviting all diabetes patients for a check-up once a year will cover this.

DM 4. Ninety percent of smokers in the diabetes group should have been offered smoking advice in the last 15 months – 5 points.

For those attending their annual review, smoking advice can be offered if they smoke, and recorded (e.g. Read code 8CAL).

DM 5. Ninety percent of diabetics should have a record of HbA_{1c} in the last 15 months – 3 points.

All diabetics should have a blood test 2 weeks before coming to the clinic. This should include either HbA_{1c} or fructosamine. When the results come into the practice they should be entered on the computer, either by lab links or manually. Patients attending the hospital clinic should have this result extracted from the clinic letter and entered manually. Read code = 42W.

DM 6. Fifty percent of diabetics should have an HbA_{1c} (or equivalent) of 7.4 or less in the last 15 months – 16 points.

This can only be achieved by tightening up on the patient's glycaemic control via diet and medication. As is well known, the target is impossible to achieve in some people. However, many other patients are only just over target, and an ethos of tightening control in this group is the strategy most likely to produce good overall results.

DM 7. Eighty-five percent of diabetics should have an HbA_{1c} (or equivalent) of 10 or less in the last 15 months – 11 points.

See above. Hopefully patients above this target are few enough to be able to be relaxed about. If they are no more than one in 10 diabetics, consider referring them to hospital for possible insulin. If they are on insulin, are they non-compliant with medication? If so, can they be excluded from the denominator for audit purposes? (See Exclusions, page 79)

DM 8. Ninety percent of diabetics should have a record of retinal screening in the past 15 months – 5 points.

Opticians now routinely perform this task. Many patients need reminding to go once a year, and this should be checked at the annual diabetes clinic. Fortunately, opticians send GPs a written report, enabling the data to be entered on the practice's computer system. Hospital diabetes clinic letters should contain the same information. There should be a line on the diabetes data grid for recording the presence or otherwise of diabetic retinopathy. Decide who is going to enter the data. Make sure everyone in the practice knows who it is. Read code = 68A7 "Diabetic retinal screening".

DM 9. Ninety percent of diabetics should have had their peripheral pulses checked and recorded in the past 15 months – 3 points.

This also forms part of the annual diabetes clinic review. A podiatrist is able to do this check. Data entry responsibility should be decided. Read codes are 24E "Pulses right" and 24F "Pulses left".

DM 10. Ninety percent of diabetics should have a record of neuropathy testing in the past 15 months – 3 points.

As above. Read code = 68A1 "Neurological screening".

DM 11. Ninety percent of diabetics should have a record of blood pressure in the past 15 months – 3 points.

Checking blood pressure should form an integral part of the annual diabetes clinic check. Correct data entry is important. For Read codes see CHD section.

DM 12. The last blood pressure reading should be 145/85 or less in 55% of diabetic patients – 17 points.

This is where the person seeing the patient needs to be able to alter the medication if necessary. A nurse could be seeing patients, referring to a doctor those with readings above 145/85 or asking for advice from a doctor at the time of the nurse consultation. Whoever takes the blood pressure should have responsibility for making sure the patient is not left for another year without further attempts to get a normal blood pressure reading onto the computer. Altering the medication, seeing the patient for follow-up, aiming for <145/85 and recording results are all essential. Remember those patients who can be excluded (see page 79).

DM 13. Ninety percent of diabetes patients should have been tested for micro-albuminuria in the last 15 months (exception reporting for proteinuria) – 3 points.

Test strips need to be purchased for testing for microalbuminuria as part of the annual diabetes clinic check-up. The Read code to use is 46W "Urine – microalbumin".

Patients known previously to have proteinuria should be checked for proteinuria annually instead.

DM 14. Ninety percent of diabetics should have had a serum creatinine result recorded in the last 15 months – 3 points.

This is easily achieved by including the test in the batch of bloods requested prior to the annual diabetic clinic. Read code = 44J3.

DM 15. Seventy percent of diabetics with proteinuria or microalbuminuria should be taking an ACE inhibitor or A_2 antagonist – 3 points.

This can be checked at the annual diabetes clinic. New cases and pre-existing cases not on this medication need to be started on treatment. The clinic nurse should discuss the case with the GP and medication started so long as there are no contraindications. Ideally, the presence of microalbuminuria should be confirmed on two further tests. If these are negative, remove all records of a positive test, as this will unfavourably skew the audit figures. Pick up patients in this group on a drugs search.

DM 16. Ninety percent of diabetes patients should have had a total cholesterol measurement recorded in the last 15 months – 3 points.

When patients are invited for their annual check-up they can be asked to attend 2 weeks beforehand to have a blood test for total cholesterol. When the results come from the lab there must be a system in place for getting them onto the computer. This is best achieved by lab links. In the absence of links, the practice should have a policy of putting all cholesterol results on the computer by a member of staff.

DM 17. The latest total cholesterol result should be 5 mmol/l or less in 60% of diabetes patients within the last 15 months – 6 points.

There is no upper age limit in the new contract for this parameter. Excluding patients above any age threshold will need to be negotiated. Until then the same applies as for blood pressure control. Titrating statin doses upwards can be done by a well-trained nurse, but the onus is on the person managing the condition to follow the patient up until they have either achieved target or reached the maximum tolerated dose. Either way, a computer entry needs to be made confirming successful completion for payment purposes and this should not be left until the next year's clinic.

DM 18. The uptake of flu vaccine should be 85% in diabetes patients – 3 points.

This can only be done between 1 September and 31 March. Patients attending for their annual diabetes check between these dates should be immunised during their check-up. Unimmunised patients seen outside this range can only be advised to have the jab next time. However, patients can be excluded from this target if they have refused or failed to attend after three invitations to do so. Sending two reminders to diabetes patients during the flu jab season is therefore important.

Reward for diabetes

A total of 99 points is available for reaching these targets. For 2004/5 this is worth an average of £6750 per 5000 patients, rising to £10,800 per 5000 patients from 2005/6.

CHRONIC OBSTRUCTIVE PULMONARY DISEASE

COPD 1. The practice can produce a register of patients with COPD – 5 points.

Simply run a search of all registered patients with any record of a Read code starting with H32 for COPD. Remember to make this a hierarchical search, i.e. to include patients with all codes beginning with H32, not just those having the H32 code in isolation. The elimination of ghost patients is crucial (see above). The true prevalence of COPD is probably as high as 16% of the population, but under-diagnosis is considerable. The important thing is to be close to your PCO average.

COPD 2. Ninety percent of patients diagnosed after 1 April 2003 should have had the diagnosis confirmed by spirometry, including reversibility testing – 5 points.

It is therefore important not to enter an H32 code until spirometry confirms the diagnosis. This is a message for those doctors who are likely to be seeing patients with suspected COPD. A better Read code to use initially will be the one that reflects the symptoms/signs, e.g. 1739 "Short of breath". Letters from hospital confirming COPD should have the Read code 33G1 "Spirometry reversibility positive" entered at the same time as the H32 code.

COPD 3. Ninety percent of all COPD patients should have had the diagnosis confirmed by spirometry, including reversibility testing – 5 points.

It is likely that most patients with a diagnosis of COPD will not have had spirometry performed. Written invitations should be extended, staged throughout the year, to ask patients to come in for spirometry and reversibility testing. This can coincide with repeat medication review. Spirometers are easily purchased for about £500 and practice nurses can be trained in their use. Patients refusing or failing to attend after three written invitations can be excluded from the denominator (see page 79).

COPD 4. Ninety percent of COPD patients should have had their smoking status recorded in the past 15 months – 6 points.

Patients with COPD will need to be invited to attend the surgery for a check-up once a year. This will include recording their smoking status. Non-responders should be excluded from the denominator. For Read codes see CHD section.

COPD 5. Ninety percent of COPD patients who smoke should have been offered smoking cessation advice in the last 15 months – 6 points.

The offer of advice can be recorded for those who are invited for their annual check-up.

COPD 6. Seventy percent of COPD patients should have had their FEV_1 recorded in the last 27 months – 6 points.

Patients should have spirometry repeated on alternate clinic attendances. If there is any doubt that the patient will return the following year, it is safer to perform spirometry annually. The Read code is 68M "Spirometry screening".

COPD 7. Ninety percent of COPD patients on inhaled therapy should have had their inhaler technique checked in the last 2 years – 6 points.

This can also be done at the annual check-up. The Read code is 6637 "Inhaler technique observed".

COPD 8. The uptake of flu vaccine should be 85% in COPD patients – 6 points.

This can only be done between 1 September and 31 March. Patients attending for their annual COPD check between these dates should be immunised during their check-up. Unimmunised patients seen outside this range can only be advised to have the jab next time. However, patients can be excluded from this target if they have refused or failed to attend after three invitations to do so. Sending two reminders to COPD patients during the flu jab season is therefore important. For Read codes see CHD section.

Reward for COPD

A total of 45 points is available for reaching these targets. For 2004/5 this is worth an average of £3068 per 5000 patients, rising to £4909 per 5000 patients from 2005/6.

Epilepsy

EPILEPSY 1. The practice can produce a register of patients receiving drug treatment for epilepsy – 2 points.

Run a search on the registered patients who are on repeat prescriptions of the group, "Drugs to control epilepsy". The numbers should be small – less than 1%. The Read code for "Epilepsy" is F25.

EPILEPSY 2. Ninety percent of epilepsy patients aged 16 and over should have a record of seizure frequency in the past 15 months – 4 points.

Write to all epilepsy patients over 15 years of age when their annual repeat prescription comes up for renewal. Ask when their last seizure occurred. Record the answer on the computer record. Preferred Read code = 6675 "Seizure frequency recorded".

EPILEPSY 3. Ninety percent of epilepsy patients aged 16 and over should have had a medication review recorded in the past 15 months – 4 points.

Remember to review medication before updating the annual repeat authorisation. Enter the Read code 667 "Epilepsy medication review".

EPILEPSY 4. Seventy percent of patients aged 16 and over on drug treatment for epilepsy should be convulsion-free for the last 12 months, recorded during the last 15 months – 6 points.

Patients declaring a seizure during the past 12 months, when asked about this in their annual letter, should be invited to come in to see the doctor to discuss altering medication. Alternatively, referral to a specialist can be arranged. It is unlikely that more than 30% of epileptics will not be well controlled.

Reward for epilepsy

A total of 16 points is available for reaching these targets. For 2004/5 this is worth an average of £1090 per 5000 patients, rising to £1746 per 5000 patients from 2005/6.

Hypothyroidism

THYROID 1. The practice can produce a register of patients with hypothyroidism – 2 points.

Run a drug search for thyroxine on repeat prescription. The prevalence should be about 1.5% and should compare well with your PCO average. Read codes are C03 "Congenital hypothyroidism" and C04 "Acquired hypothyroidism".

THYROID 2. Ninety percent of patients with hypothyroidism should have had their TFTs recorded within the last 15 months – 6 points.

Authorise thyroxine on repeat prescription for 1 year. When the repeat comes around for renewal, send the patient an invitation to come in for a blood test for TSH. Update the prescription for a further month. When updating the repeats that have been authorised for 1 month only, check to see if a TSH has been recorded. If so, update the repeats for a further year. If not, update for 1 month and send a further reminder. TSH results should be entered on the computer by a member of staff, or by lab links, if available. Read code = 442.

Reward for hypothyroidism

Eight points are available for reaching these targets. For 2004/5 this is worth an average of £545 per 5000 patients, rising to £873 per 5000 patients from 2005/6.

CANCER

CANCER 1. The practice can produce a register of all cancer patients, defined as "a register of patients with a diagnosis of cancer excluding non-melanotic skin cancers from 1 April 2003" – 6 points.

Choose a Read code that will be used to define this group, say Read code B "Neoplasms". Use this as a marker for all new diagnoses since 1 April 2003. Alternatively, run a hierarchical search on Read code B, excluding B33 for skin cancers, and then manually adding back any malignant melanomas that had been incorrectly coded as B33 (instead of B32).

CANCER 2. Ninety percent of patients with cancer diagnosed since 1 April 2003 should have had a review by the practice, to include an assessment of support needs and co-ordination with secondary care, within 6 months of diagnosis – 6 points.

Patients fulfilling this requirement should have a Read code 8CL0 "Cancer diagnosis discussed" entered on their clinical record. Existing patients will be known to the GP or district nurse. Unknown patients appearing in the search should be invited for review if appropriate. If the patient has no need for further involvement, the Read code 8CL0 should be entered to show that the patient's needs have been reviewed.

Reward for cancer

A total of 12 points is available for reaching these targets. For 2004/5 this is worth an average of £818 per 5000 patients, rising to £1309 per 5000 patients from 2005/6.

MENTAL HEALTH

MH 1. The practice can produce a register of people with severe long-term mental health problems who require and have agreed to regular follow-up – 7 points.

By definition, this group of patients should be having regular appointments with specialist services. They include people with schizophrenia and manic depression. Search on Read codes E10 "Schizophrenic disorders" and E11 "Affective psychoses". Exclude Read codes E118 "Seasonal affective disorder" and E112 "Single major depressive episode". Patients who should be on the register can be given the Read code 9H8 "Mental health register", and this code used in future to simplify searching.

MH 2. Ninety percent of patients in the above group should have had a review in the previous 15 months. This includes a check on the accuracy of prescribed medication, a review of physical health and a review of co-ordination arrangements with secondary care – 23 points.

Review the records of the above group. Letters from their psychiatrist should confirm that the above review has been undertaken. Most should have been seen at least annually. Patients on the disease register who have not been reviewed should either be removed from the register (e.g. due to misdiagnosis, low severity) or be referred for specialist review. There is no exact Read code to record this activity, but 8B3S "Medication review" has been chosen as the preferred coding by the BMA/DoH.

MH 3. Ninety percent of patients on lithium therapy should have a record of lithium levels checked within the last 6 months – 3 points.

Run a drug search on lithium. Check the records for lithium levels. Ring the lab if the bloods are monitored in secondary care. Enter the latest result on the computer under Read code 44W8.11 "Lithium: blood level". Lithium patients should be encouraged to have blood testing every 3 months and the results should be entered on the computer, either manually or via lab links if available. Patients' repeat pre-scriptions should be authorised for 6 months. On updating the repeat, check that the bloods have been done. If not, send the patient a reminder and update the repeat for just 1 month. After that month, check for a result again. Update for 6 months if there is a result, 1 month if not. Read code = 44W8.

MH 4. Ninety percent of patients on lithium therapy should have a record of serum creatinine and TSH in the preceding 15 months – 3 points.

These can be included in the lithium blood test. Preferred coding is: 442 "Thyroid function tests" and 44J3 "Serum creatinine".

MH 5. Seventy percent of patients on lithium therapy should have a result within the therapeutic range within the previous 6 months – 5 points.

Contact patients outside the therapeutic range to check on compliance and/or to adjust the dosage as appropriate. Repeat the bloods after 1 month.

Reward for mental health

A total of 41 points is available for reaching these targets. For 2004/5 this is worth an average of £2796 per 5000 patients, rising to £4473 per 5000 patients from 2005/6.

ASTHMA

ASTHMA 1. The practice can produce a register of patients with asthma, excluding patients with asthma who have been prescribed no asthma-related drugs in the last 12 months – 7 points.

Run a combined search looking for patients with Read code H33 "Asthma" and those on repeat prescriptions for any of the three groups: bronchodilators, inhaled corticosteroids, and cromoglycate and leukotriene receptor antagonists. The result should be between 6.5% and 7.5% of the whole practice population. Check with the PCO that your results are consistent with theirs.

ASTHMA 2. Seventy percent of patients aged 8 and over diagnosed with asthma since 1 April 2003 should have had the diagnosis confirmed with either spirometry or peak flow measurement – 15 points.

This is a message for doctors making the diagnosis of asthma. Peak flow reversibility of at least 15% improvement after inhaled salbutamol is essential. Record the Read code 3395 "Peak flow rate abnormal" (or 33G1 if using spirometry). Enter this code on existing patient records if their peak flow diaries confirm a pre- and post-inhaler difference of 15% or more. Put a line in the computer data grid for asthma to enable easy prompting and recording of the 3395 code.

ASTHMA 3. Seventy percent of patients with asthma between the ages of 14 and 19 should have a record of smoking status in the previous 15 months – 6 points.

All asthmatics should be invited to attend the surgery for an annual check-up. Reminders can be sent out with their repeat prescriptions, with repeat updates limited to 1 month at a time until the patient is seen. Thereafter, the repeats can be re-authorised for 1 year. The data grid for asthma should contain a line for smoking status (Read code 137 "Tobacco consumption"). For Read codes see CHD section.

ASTHMA 4. Seventy percent of asthmatics aged 20 and over should have a record of smoking status in the previous 15 months, unless they are recorded as non-smokers – 6 points.

As above.

ASTHMA 5. Seventy percent of asthmatic smokers should have been offered smoking cessation advice within the previous 15 months – 6 points.

The data grid for asthma management should contain a line for smoking cessation advice offered (Read code 8CAL). The advice can be offered to patients as they are invited for their asthma check-up.

ASTHMA 6. Seventy percent of patients with asthma should have had an asthma review within the previous 15 months – 20 points.

Tying in the invitation for an annual asthma check with the repeat prescription allows a cheap, effective and direct means of communication with the patient, which can be monitored each month. A letter of invitation is generally better than a rubber stamp. Read code = 66YJ "Asthma review".

ASTHMA 7. Seventy percent of asthma patients aged 16 and over should have had a flu jab during the previous winter – 12 points.

This can only be given between 1 September and 31 March. Patients attending for their annual asthma check between these dates should be immunised during their check-up. Unimmunised patients seen outside this range can only be advised to have the jab next time. However, patients can be excluded from this target if they have refused or failed to attend after three invitations to do so. Sending two reminders to asthma patients during the flu jab season is therefore important.

Reward for asthma

A total of 72 points is available for reaching these targets. For 2004/5 this is worth an average of £4909 per 5000 patients, rising to £7855 per 5000 patients from 2005/6.

SUMMARY OF CLINICAL QUALITY MARKERS

A total of 550 points is available for achieving the maximum targets in all clinical areas. The highest target in any area is 90%, allowing one in 10 patients to fall through the net. The maximum targets are attainable with well-resourced, well-organised care.

The total maximum rewards for an average practice of 5000 patients are:

£37,500 for 2004/5
£60,000 for 2005/6

Clearly, this more than covers the cost of employing a full-time additional practice nurse, whose sole responsibility would be to achieve the maximum clinical targets in all areas.

ORGANISATIONAL QUALITY INDICATORS

There are five categories of organisational indicator and a total of 56 indicators. All indicators are of the Yes/No type. Note that some indicators appear to repeat others. This is a device to permit different levels of achievement.

A. RECORDS AND INFORMATION ABOUT PATIENTS – 85 POINTS

Essentially this can only be achieved in fully computerised practices, where all patient contacts and prescribing are recorded on the computer. Other practice organisational systems, such as message books, visit books, in-trays for lab results and hospital letters, and mechanisms for communicating with the out-of-hours service, are already commonplace in nearly every practice.

The areas to focus on are:

- Summarising notes of existing patients, and new patients within 8 weeks.

- Recording a clinical indication for all new drugs added to the repeat prescription screen.

- Regular, opportunistic recording of smoking status and blood pressure on existing patients.

B. Patient communication – 8 points

These 8 points can all be achieved by having:

- A practice leaflet.

- Opening hours of at least 9 a.m. to 6 p.m. Monday to Friday.

- Call divert for directing patient telephone calls to the out-of-hours service after hours.

- A smoke-stop strategy.

- A policy of how to remove patients from the list.

C. Education and training – 29 points

This essentially refers to the presence of a policy on:

- Annual appraisal of all staff.

- Basic life-support training.

- Critical incident/significant event analysis.

- A complaints policy.

The actual details are easily achieved if these processes are in place. The practice manager should be able to ensure these points are easily earned.

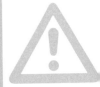

MANAGER'S TIP

SIGNIFICANT EVENT ANALYSIS (SEA)

Set up a system that is:

· User-friendly, i.e. the recording mechanism is easy to use and readily accessible.

· Non-threatening. SEA is about learning how we can do things better. It is not about pointing fingers and allocating blame.

Develop a simple pro forma (either manual or electronic) to capture the following data:

· What happened to make this a significant event, e.g. what went wrong.

· How did it affect:
  – The individual team member
  – The practice as a whole
  – The patient.

· What lessons have been learnt.

· How can you stop it happening again.

· What is the action plan.

Review significant events regularly at Primary Health Care Team meetings and reflect on the outcomes. This should be a positive experience. You can't change what has already happened but you can influence the future.

N.B. Significant events analysis can also include things that went well in unusual circumstances, e.g. the way in which the team dealt with a death in the treatment room.

D. PRACTICE MANAGEMENT – 20 POINTS

This broad category of organisational markers covers some of the usual roles of the practice manager, such as:

• Computer back-up.

• Job descriptions for staff.

- Fraud prevention.

- Employment policies.

Others to check on are:

- Hepatitis B status of all personnel.

- Provision of a copy of the local child protection policy.

- Instrument sterilisation.

- Instrument maintenance and calibration.

- Information for carers.

E. Medicines management – 42 points

Assuming the prescribing system is computerised, there are essentially three categories.

- Efficient turnaround of repeats and annual review of medication recorded upon re-authorising further annual repeats (Read code 8BI).

- Taking part in project work with the local prescribing adviser.

- Emergency and other black bag drugs well maintained.

Summary of organisational quality indicators

The total number of points available for organisational quality is 184. For the average practice of 5000 patients, this is worth:

£12,546 for 2004/5
£20,073 for 2005/6

The extra work involved in achieving this should be minimal in a well-run practice. There may be a need to employ a notes summariser and there are also a number of one-off policies to put in place initially. Practice managers should be able to develop the systems to achieve these targets easily.

PATIENT EXPERIENCE

Patient experience indicators comprise two categories: length of consultations and the patient survey. Indicators are of the Yes/No type. Note that the patient survey indicator has three levels to permit different levels of achievement.

1. LENGTH OF CONSULTATIONS — 30 POINTS

If your practice already runs to 10-minute appointments, these 30 points are a giveaway. Practices that run to 10 minutes but with extras in the middle should think about listing the extras at the beginning or end of the booked appointments.

Practices with open appointments or 5/7.5-minute appointments could consider running longer surgeries, employing extra doctors, cutting down on other work (that may be worth less than these 30 points) or closing their lists.

Thirty points are worth £2046 in 2004/5, increasing to £3273 in 2005/6 for the average list of 5000 patients.

2. PATIENT SURVEYS — 70 POINTS

Two different patient surveys have been approved by the NHS Confederation and the BMA for the purpose of achieving the patient experience quality marker. They are (see Appendix 4):

- General Practice Assessment Questionnaire (GPAQ), developed by the National Primary Care Research and Development Centre in Manchester.

- Improving Practice Questionnaire (IPQ), developed by Exeter University.

Implementing the outcome of the survey is at the discretion of the practice. It is not essential to establish a patient group. The practice manager should be able to co-ordinate the work, discussing the patients' comments at a practice meeting. Involve the PCO by sending them the results and inviting their comments.

ADDITIONAL SERVICES (ADDITIONAL PAYMENTS FOR QUALITY)

There are four categories of additional services indicator and a total of 10 indicators. All are of the Yes/No type except the first, which requires a percentage to be entered and for which achievement is calculated in the same way as for clinical indicators.

1. Cervical screening – 22 points

These points are earned by continuing to perform adequate cervical smears on at least 80% of eligible women, for auditing inadequate smears and for informing women of their smear results.

2. Child health surveillance – 6 points

Running the baby clinic to local guidelines and following up problems is worth 6 points – £409 per year for the average practice of 5000 patients in 2004/5. This does not include payments for childhood immunisations (£2941 for additional services plus directed enhanced service payment for higher target achievement) nor payment for running the CHS service as an additional service (£2106 per 5000 average population for 2004/5).

3. Maternity services – 6 points

Compliance with local guidelines is worth 6 points.

4. Contraceptive services – 2 points

A written policy for emergency contraception and pre-conceptual counselling are all that are required. Other contraception services are paid for via the additional services payment of £7383 per 5000 average patients for 2004/5.

Holistic care payments

One hundred extra points are available for achieving high quality across all the clinical quality areas. The third-lowest scoring disease area dictates the level of holistic care payment. In other words, you need to monitor your progress throughout the year, putting most effort into whichever disease area is currently scoring third from bottom in your league table. If that was, say, hypothyroidism, improving the score in that disease would be worth far more than the 8 points normally assigned to it.

Furthermore, if you decide you cannot hope to score highly on all diseases, then don't neglect more than two; otherwise, your holistic care payment will be hit hard.

Quality practice payment

This is worth 30 points and is awarded in the same way as the holistic care payment, except that it rewards overall achievement across all the non-clinical areas.

The same advice applies here, in that most effort should be applied near the bottom of the league table for your practice.

ACCESS

Practices able to meet the national access targets can receive an additional 50 points, taking the total available to 1050. See the seperate chapter on Access for further details on how to achieve access targets.

Manipulating appointments can achieve the same end so far as the access points are concerned. By making some appointments book-on-the-day only, patients who request an appointment within 48 hours can often be accommodated.

RISING UP THE QUALITY LADDER

The payments for quality are high and there is a linear increase in payments the higher you get. Practices may feel they have reached their natural ceiling in rising up the quality ladder and that further improvements would mean an unacceptable extra effort. This feeling should be resisted. Achieving the maximum target payment is possible.

Monitoring progress across the different areas in an accurate, regular and considered way will help to highlight those areas where higher targets may have been narrowly missed. Improving the achievement in those areas will earn more points than slavishly pursuing other targets that may need more work; that can come later.

Improving in the third-lowest-scoring clinical and organisational areas will bring double the rewards by earning points for holistic care payments or quality practice payments.

It may be that extra achievement will need more investment in nursing/staff hours. The cost of this is well worth it due to the high value of the payment per point. What might seem like an insurmountable task will feel within sight when the hours are there to enable taking on the work.

Have an ethos of improvement. Aim for annual increases in quality achievements and payments. Involve the whole team and create a sense of pride in striving for 1050 points for your practice.

Troubleshooting

Missing a target does not mean the end of the world. In fact, it doesn't matter if you fail to reach the targets you have already received aspiration payments for; the achievement payments will be reduced to compensate.

Have a no-blame culture in your practice. Look at where targets have been missed and by how much. Ask why they were missed and learn from it. Use the quality management team in your practice to analyse the findings and make recommendations to the practice.

Having said that, it sometimes helps to analyse the results in groups by clinician. The identification of one or two doctors or nurses who keep forgetting to tick the right box can be effectively dealt with by circulating everybody's results around the whole team for comparison. Consistent under-performance is letting down the whole practice and eating into profitability. If there are still difficulties getting data recorded, ask the person why. Could there be a better way of entering the data? An example might be the use of a data grid in hard copy.

Computer glitches should be ironed out as early as possible. Comparing audit/search results with a sample of individual patient records will highlight inaccuracies in Read coding and search set-up. Close monitoring at regular intervals will pick this up. Remember to use the advice line of the medical system supplier for difficult problems. The chances are there are other practices with similar problems.

Other useful sources of advice include:

- Medical Audit Advisory Group, if there is one in your area.

- Primary Care Organisation.

- Practice managers' group.

- Your own staff.

ENHANCED SERVICES

INTRODUCTION

Enhanced services are the truly optional part of NHS general practice. Unlike essential services, which are, as the name suggests, an inescapable element of the GMS contract, and additional services, which most practices provide, the enhanced element has the private medicine advantage of being a valuable source of optional extra income.

There are several reasons for wanting to set up a contract to provide an enhanced service: clinical interest, local need, pre-existing provision. But before leaping into a commitment to your PCO you will need to examine it under the bright light of the "financeoscope".

FINANCES

This book is unashamedly about making a healthy profit in general practice. When a practice decides to offer extra services to its patients (and, in the case of some of the enhanced services, also to patients of other practices), it has to perform a financial analysis.

- What is the contract price for the service in question?

- What will the workload be, and who will do the work?

- What other services may suffer as a result of taking on the new service?

- What are the training, infrastructure and on-costs?

- Is the future funding of the service secure?

The answers to these questions feed into a complex and fuzzy formula, which should be picked apart by the financial brains of the practice. The outcome, however, will be a straightforward yes or no. Either we go for it or we don't, and, if our decision is correct, then we will have taken another step closer to achieving maximum profitability for the practice.

Accountant's tip

GPs have a financial choice to make. This is called "opportunity costing". Do you undertake further enhanced services or do you spend your time more lucratively on other work? Apart from the income, you must consider the costs, which might include staffing, nursing, external technical costs, deputising and drug costs.

It is important not to cloud the analysis with bogus arguments.

- Are there risks associated with the service (litigation, violent attack)?

- Do we have the skills?

- Do we like that sort of medicine?

- Can we be bothered?

- Will it make me look good in the eyes of my colleagues/PCO/patients?

- Will it get me out of doing routine surgeries?

If the service is worth pursuing financially then other obstacles should be tackled and resolved.

Types of service

There are three types of enhanced service: directed, national and local.

Directed enhanced services

These are extra services that are outside the remit of essential and additional services, that the PCO must provide and that have a nationally negotiated specification and price. They include:

- Provision for seeing violent patients.

- Improved access.

- Childhood immunisation targets.

- Influenza immunisation.

- Quality information preparation.

- Advanced minor surgery (beyond simple cautery for skin lesions).

Practices will already have considerable expertise and infrastructure to provide many of these services. Have a close dialogue with your PCO about which services you can offer to them, not only for your patients but for those of other practices. These services are entirely optional and there may be doctors in your area who would rather not try to provide them. Remember, therefore, when setting the contract specifications, to state the volume of work/number of patients involved.

MANAGER'S TIP

As with any dialogue with your PCO, make sure that you are talking to those who are in a position to negotiate with you and to make decisions! Valuable time (and money) is wasted when decision-making has to be referred backwards and forwards to other committees. Equally, those representing the practice must also be in a position to make decisions.

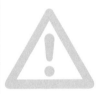

If your practice already provides these services, the training and infrastructure costs will be minimised and the running costs should be well known, and so the decision on future provision will hinge largely on the contract price.

NATIONAL ENHANCED SERVICES

These are like directed enhanced services in that their specification and price are negotiated nationally, but unlike directed services they are not mandatory for PCOs. These services may have been provided by secondary care or other providers within the NHS or social services. Examples include:

- Intra-partum care.

- Anticoagulant monitoring.

- IUCD fitting.

- Drug and alcohol misuse services.

- Specialised sexual health services.

- Specialised depression services.

- Multiple sclerosis services.

- Enhanced care of the homeless.

- Immediate care and first response care.

- Minor injury services.

- Near-patient testing.

If your practice currently provides these services, make sure you get the opportunity to be paid for them via a national enhanced services contract. Doctors in rural and remote areas will be asked by their PCO to continue to provide services in this way.

If you don't currently provide these services, look at the service specifications to see if you could provide the services at a profit. Remember, you can buy in the medical/nursing expertise to provide the work and use the practice simply as an administrative tool and contract-holder. A predatory approach towards the PCO is more likely to secure a contract. The PCO's vulnerabilities lie in their enormous workload, relative lack of clinical input, obligations to the Department of Health and need for cost-effectiveness. All these pressures can be exploited when presenting your case to the PCO.

LOCAL ENHANCED SERVICES

These are extra services that practices may provide that are outside the remit of essential and additional services, and that are negotiated locally between the practice and the PCO. They may include such things as:

- Cover for a local cottage hospital.

- The provision of additional services to an opted-out practice.

- Running an adolescent health clinic at a local school.

- Continuing to provide Saturday morning surgeries after December 2004.

- Nursing home cover.

- Community psychiatric care.

- Anything else you do outside essential and additional services that does not attract a private fee.

If you are already providing these services, make sure you tell your PCO. Work out how much it costs you to provide a service, and decide whether you want to continue to provide it or not. Fix the price by negotiation with the PCO; their need for you to continue doing the work will dictate how hard you can drive up the price. If there is no alternative provider you should take a hard line. Don't listen to their pleas for clemency, and certainly don't agree to do the work "to help out the NHS". Remember, enhanced services are optional under the GMS contract. If the price is not appealing, just say no!

MANAGER'S TIP

Never undersell yourself. How much could you attract by letting accommodation to commercial tenants, e.g. chiropractor, aromatherapist or someone independently undertaking medico-legal work? Remember, price is driven by traditional supply and demand economics.

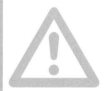

EXAMPLES

Influenza immunisations
This is a service that has traditionally been provided in general practice, and there is an expectation among patients that this will remain the case. However, as an enhanced service, any practice is free to return this obligation to their PCO.

Income
A fee of £6.80 in 2003/4 is payable to practices for every patient given a flu jab if they are in a high-risk group. This figure will rise to £7.02 for 2004/5.

- Aged 65 and over.

- Living in long-stay facilities, e.g. nursing/residential homes.

- Chronic respiratory disease including all asthmatics.

- Chronic heart disease.

- Chronic renal disease.

- Immunocompromise.

- Diabetes mellitus.

In addition to the direct income for giving flu jabs, there is income from achieving higher targets under the quality and outcomes (Q&O) scheme for CHD, asthma, COPD, stroke/TIA and diabetes mellitus. If all the targets for flu jabs are reached, the Q&O scheme income for the average practice of 5000 patients is £2046 for 2004/5 and £3273 for 2005/6, assuming the average practice of 5000 patients has 1500 patients eligible for the flu jab, of whom 1000 also have one of the conditions in the Q&O scheme.

Let's also assume that the practice will be doing well if it immunises 70% of all those who are eligible.

The income for 2004/5 will be:

Enhanced service income	70% of 1500 x £7.02	= £7371
Quality points income	26.83 points x £75	= £2012
Total income		= £9383

The costs will be:

Supply of 1150 flu vaccines, including discount and surplus stock	= £4436
Nursing time at £20 per hour (total cost to employer)	= £600
Administration time at £10 per hour (ditto)	= £100
Total expenses	= **5136**
Profit to practice	= **4247**

For dispensing practices there will also be dispensing payments of approximately £8468 on 1050 vaccines prescribed.

CALCULATED PROFIT VS ACTUAL PROFIT: THE DIFFERENCES

Using employed staff to run a service such as flu immunisation does have financial costs for the practice. These costs should therefore be included in the calculations when looking at expanding into new services and when comparing one new service with another.

In reality, however, it is unusual to have to take on extra nurses to provide flu jabs and, in many practices, this extra seasonal work is absorbed into the nurses' and other staff members' normal working hours.

Imagine, though, that you were thinking of abandoning flu jabs, perhaps because you felt they were unprofitable or excessively bureaucratic. Would you be able to cut your nurses' hours as a result? If not, then those staff costs remain in the practice balance sheet and must either be met out of existing income or used to generate alternative new income.

In short, both the profits from continuing to provide an existing service and, conversely, the loss of profit from abandoning an existing service, are greater than the calculations suggest.

THE WORKFORCE SPONGE: ECONOMIES OF SCALE

Expanding a service like flu immunisation to include patients of other practices brings in extra income for little additional expenditure. With the infrastructure, training and administration already established, the nurses' time is the only extra cost to be met. Vaccine costs reduce as volume increases, due to discounts and the diluting of surplus stock over a larger patient field.

The practice's workforce can usually take on more of the same sort of work without a proportionate increase in disruption, costs and administrative turmoil. Take on enough nursing hours and your practice could immunise all the patients in the county!

DIVERSITY

In reality, however, very few practices are likely to release their own patients into the flu vaccination market. But what of the other enhanced services?

Which services are unlikely to be provided by most practices? In view of the fact that there has been a vocalisation of GPs' discontent with some aspects of their work, one might conclude that there will be scope to provide services on behalf of the whole PCO.

Examples might be:

- Violent patients.

- Alcohol misuse.

- Drug misuse.

- IUCD fitting.

- Homeless.

- Intra-partum care.

- Community in-patient care.

- Specialised minor surgery.

- Other specialist services that the PCO wishes to provide.

GPs who already provide such services will be at an advantage when tendering to widen their provision to other practices or the whole PCO. Professional expertise, premises, staff, supplies and administration will already be established. Furthermore, the reputation of a local doctor as a provider of a specialist service will carry a certain amount of weight in the PCO.

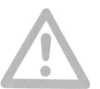

MANAGER'S TIP

Be prepared to invest in training for areas you wish to develop. (If you don't, someone else will fill that gap and attract the income.)

Training in these areas is readily available to all doctors, through the Royal Colleges or from local secondary care services. For example, a course is available from the Royal College of General Practitioners for training GPs in the management of drug abuse. A diploma recognises specialist skills and will almost certainly be a requirement of new providers of some of these enhanced services.

GPs hoping to fill practice vacancies could make themselves more marketable by arming themselves with those diplomas that can earn a practice extra income through enhanced services.

THE ENHANCED SERVICES: HOW MUCH ARE THEY WORTH?

DIRECTED ENHANCED SERVICES

1. Access (see chapter on Access)

In general, this requires the practice to be able to give a patient an appointment with a GP within 48 hours.

A sum of £5000 is payable in 2003/4 per 5500 patients if the standard is met. Half the money is paid in advance, the remainder on completion of a successful year. In addition, 50 Quality points are payable, worth £3750 per 5500 patients in 2003/4 and £6000 in 2004/5.

2. Childhood immunisations

Immunising 90% of all the practice's 2- and 5-year-old children is worth a total of £10,430 for an average list of 5000 patients in 2003/4, increasing to £10,766 in 2004/5 and £11,114 in 2005/6. Opting out of providing this service will also cost the practice 1% of its global sum.

ACCOUNTANT'S TIP

Childhood immunisations are very important and should not be overlooked. Opting out will cost the practice dearly.

3. Influenza

See above example.

4. Quality information preparation

A total of £5000 per 5500 patients is available to be spent on clinical notes summarising. This sum is only meant to be available if the practice needs to summarise. Claim your need.

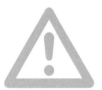

MANAGER'S TIP

Even if you think your summaries are fully computerised, changes in computer systems, variable use of Read codes and changes in practice personnel might have left a few gaps that need to be tidied up to ensure the quality of your data.

5. Violent patients

This payment is for providing essential and additional services for patients who have been struck off a practice's list for violent behaviour. The payments for providing the service in 2003/4 are:

Retainer fee	£2000 per annum
Consultation fee	£40–80 (in-hours)
Infrastructure	£2500 per annum

The annual increases are 3.225%.

6. Minor surgery

Included in the practice's global sum is a payment for simple cautery. Opting out of providing this will cost the practice approximately £600 per GP. Providing minor surgery above this standard will attract extra payments. These range from £150 for a session of joint injections, through £250 for surgery such as toenail removal, excision biopsy, etc., to £350 for a session of vasectomies/varicose vein surgery.

The exact number of procedures/sessions is negotiated with the PCO and will depend on whether the practice performs surgery on the patients of other practices. Contracts are either block contracts or cost and volume contracts.

A block contract involves a predetermined annual payment for all the surgery the practice does under that contract, irrespective of the number of procedures. A cost and volume contract pays a set price for all the procedures up to a set number and then an additional item of service payment for all procedures above that number.

NATIONAL ENHANCED SERVICES

1. Alcohol misuse service

This requires the practice to offer home detoxification as well as referral to and liaison with specialist services.

A retainer fee of £1000 per practice per annum for 2003/4 is payable. In addition, £200 per patient on the alcohol register is paid. These figures are up-rated by 3.225% per year.

2. Anticoagulation monitoring

Four levels of payment are available per anticoagulated patient per year in 2003/4:

£6–10	where the haematology lab does all the routine work
£75–100	where the practice does the dosing
£80–110	where the practice also funds the phlebotomist
£85–120	where the practice also measures the INR

With, say, 70 patients on warfarin, the average practice sending samples to the lab but doing their own dosing would earn about £7000 a year.

3. Fitting coils

This also covers the use of progestogen IUS for menorrhagia.

The fee in 2003/4 is £75 per insertion and £20 per annual check-up, rising by 3.225% per year.

4. Specialist depression services

Patients diagnosed as depressed by a specialist can be cared for in general practice for an additional fee. Maintaining a patient's personal health plan, liaising with secondary care and using accredited monitoring questionnaires are all part of the contract requirements.

The fees are:

£1000 retainer per practice for 2003/4
£80–100 per patient per year

5. Drug misuse service

Assessing drug use, identifying problems, prescribing maintenance and withdrawal regimes, and liaising with specialist services are all involved in the contract.

The fees are:

> £1000 retainer per practice per year in 2003/4
> £500 per patient for withdrawal
> £350 per patient per year for maintenance prescribing

6. Immediate and first response care

PCOs offer this contract to GPs in rural and remote areas of the UK. Doctors need to hold a pre-hospital emergency medicine qualification and work closely with the ambulance services.

The fees payable are:

> £1200–1500 annual retainer per practice for 2003/4
> £60–90 per in-hours call-out
> £120–150 per out-of-hours call-out

7. Care of the homeless

For practices in areas with sufficient numbers of homeless people, this enhanced service will be worth considering. Essentially, the practice has to provide essential and additional services to people with no fixed abode and to liaise with a local pharmacy to facilitate single daily dosing of drugs.

The fees are:

> £1000 annual retainer for 2003/4
> £100 per patient

8. Intra-partum care

For delivering babies, either at home or in a delivery suite to reasonable defined standards of care, the fees are:

> £200 per patient
> £50 per neonatal check

9. Minor injury services

For treating injuries and wounds under 48 hours old, GPs are paid:

£1000 annual retainer in 2003/4

£50 per patient episode

If a contract for this enhanced service is not forthcoming from the PCO, then patients with such injuries should be directed to the nearest minor injuries unit/casualty department. In some areas there may be patient dissatisfaction with this arrangement. If so, a patient information leaflet should be prepared, outlining the practice's reasons for turning them away and pointing out that the PCO has the power and the means to provide a practice-based service.

10. Specialised sexual health services

For effectively running a GUM clinic the practice will be paid:

£2000 annual retainer

£100 per patient (£200 if HIV-positive)

11. Multiple sclerosis service

For the practice to provide a lead contact/co-ordinator (usually the GP) the practice will be paid:

£90–140 per annum per patient in 2003/4

12. Near-patient testing

For monitoring disease-modifying anti-rheumatoid drugs, the practice is paid the same as for anticoagulant monitoring. The number of patients is likely to be considerably smaller than for warfarin, probably around 10 per average practice of 5000.

ACCOUNTANT'S TIP

Consider your advertising. Practice leaflets should now be very explicit as to the services provided. Consider using the practice website or even Yellow Pages.

PERSONAL MEDICAL SERVICES (PMS)

At the time of writing, approximately one third of UK GPs are providing services to the NHS under PMS contracts. The new GMS contract has more in common with PMS than did the old GMS contract, but still there are many reasons for considering switching.

One of the most compelling reasons is to maintain an upward movement in practice income. NHS fees under the new GMS contract may be threatened year-on-year by the loss of medical manpower, the underachieving of quality targets and the erosion of traditional GP services by the establishment of competing service providers in the locality.

There have been five waves of PMS pilots, with 5b going live in October 2003. Before considering making an expression of interest to your PCO, remember that the baseline PMS contract price is based on the previous year's GMS income. It makes sense, therefore, to maximise GMS income before negotiating on PMS. Choosing a good year is essential, as, under PMS, all future contract values are based in this baseline GMS year.

ACCOUNTANT'S TIP

If it appears that GMS profits are threatened under the new contract, consider PMS now. Remember, however, that PMS contracts are locally negotiated with the PCO. There is no national protection.

The PMS financial contract is arrived at as follows.

1. The Health Authority produce a spreadsheet which lists a whole year's GMS (recent). This is known as the GMS baseline.

2. The spreadsheet continues sideways to include exceptional items, which cover reasons why the GMS baseline would have been altered in the future had the practice remained in GMS. Examples might be:

- A partner reaching a new level of seniority.

- A new housing estate being built and the knock-on effect on the allocation formula.

- The patient profile may be varying depending upon demography, so increasing the Carr–Hill weighting and numbers of patients in quality targets.

- Anything else you can think of.

3. The spreadsheet continues sideways to include an uplift which deals with pay awards from the GMS baseline to the introduction of the PMS contract.

4. The spreadsheet continues sideways to summate the GMS baseline plus exceptional items plus uplift, to arrive at a base PMS contract, which is then summated after adjustments are made to superannuation arising out of any of the above points.

5. Then comes one of the most important issues. To the base total is added growth funding, which is monies provided to PMS GPs for providing additional services. These services could be almost anything, provided that the Health Authority agrees that they are essential for the local area. Such services may already be provided but not paid for under GMS or they may be partly reimbursed as enhanced services.

6. The growth monies are added to the PMS base total to arrive at the PMS contract sum, which is paid to the practice on a monthly basis.

Given the above framework, the tips for negotiating a good contract must be as follows.

- Make sure the Health Authority selects a good GMS baseline. It won't help if they select a poor year. In a nutshell, maximise GMS before you embark upon PMS. Compare your figures to the national average and to your accountant's client average.

- Consider exceptional items very carefully. This involves forecasting your GMS income after the baseline to take account of all opportunities in the local area. The comparison to national average should help to identify those parts of GMS that are low.

- Make sure supperannuation is altered properly in light of the exceptional items – errors are common!

- The key is growth funding, otherwise you are unlikely to be better off. Here, negotiating skills are critical. It is no surprise that those GPs involved in their local PCO seem to negotiate better contracts.

- Make sure you have considered all services you have provided, do provide and will provide, that hitherto may not have been paid for under GMS. Services can include anything you might think of, e.g. vasectomy clinics. Growth funding might be a direct fee for the work. Alternatively, if the work takes up GP time, then a salaried GP might be provided at full reimbursement. If extra members of staff are required they may attract reimbursement in the form of growth funding. GPs have to think laterally and play themselves up. Even improving access may attract growth funding. The list is endless.

- Do not be afraid to seek professional help. At the end of the day, it is all about the provision of services that the local PCO deems to be appropriate for the locality – state and prove your case.

SOURCES OF ADVICE

- Your accountant should be the first port of call. If you are with an accountant with little or no experience of PMS, contact the Association of Independent Specialist Medical Accountants (AISMA), 48 St Leonards Road, Bexhill On Sea TN40 1JB. Tel.: 01424 730345

- Pricare, 64 Knightsbridge, London SW1X 7JF. Tel.: 0207 590 3120; e-mail: contact@pricare.co.uk

- NHS Executive website, www.doh.gov.uk

- The Regional Offices of the Department of Health also have key people to contact about PMS

- Your PCO should be approached early for an informal discussion on the support they can offer.

MAKING THE PROPOSAL

A proposal pro forma can be downloaded from the NHS Primary Care website: www.doh.gov.uk/pmsdevelopment/index.htm. Alternatively, ask your PCO to provide one.

Think carefully about why you want to become a PMS provider and elaborate on these ideals in your proposal. Don't be afraid to state that the poor income you receive from GMS is a disincentive for the future recruitment of GPs to your practice. One of the government's aims in setting up PMS was to solve the recruitment crisis in general practice.

Other NHS ideals to consider include:

- A focus on public health.

- Help for deprived/vulnerable groups.

- Closer working with social care.

- Better access.

- Wider range of services, especially from secondary care.

- Better use of GPs skills.

- Innovative use of the primary health care team.

- PCO-wide proposals.

Remember to stress the benefits of the new flexibilities to the practice, the patients, the doctors and the NHS. Using a consultancy such as Pricare is very likely to maximise the chances of your PMS proposal being accepted by the Secretary of State for Health, whose office makes the final decision on whether you proceed or not.

THE FINANCIAL BENEFITS

Under the old GMS contract, GPs who switched to PMS were, on average, about 10% better off in terms of profit share. Since then there has been considerable convergence between the new GMS contract and PMS. Quality payments are now common to both, although not by the same mechanism. Out-of-hours will be optional for both. Both contracts are practice based as opposed to individual doctor based for GMS.

The financial benefits of switching to PMS lie in security, with the contract price being negotiated and fixed in advance, rather than based on projected performance on the quality targets. There is also the possibility of negotiating payment for work outside the GMS contract, i.e. extra tasks undertaken by the practice that do not form part of an enhanced services contract at present.

Factors that increase practice workload that are not accounted for under the Carr–Hill formula for calculating the global sum, may be taken into account when negotiating the PMS baseline. These include:

- The diseconomies of scale that adversely affect small practices.

- High morbidity from uncounted conditions such as osteoarthritis.

- The higher cost of running a practice in a city other than London.

- Any other area in which you feel you have been unfairly dealt with by the GMS allocation formula.

Finally, the PMS contract price is arrived at by negotiation with the PCO. By getting expert help in doing this and by being closely involved with the PCO beforehand, the final figure can still be better than with GMS.

If there is a disappointing conclusion to PMS proposal negotiations, then the practice can pull out and remain in GMS. Even if the practice goes ahead with a PMS pilot, there is a guaranteed return ticket that can be exercised at any time by giving the PCO 6 months' notice.

SWITCHING BACK TO GMS FROM PMS

This option can be exercised at any time, giving 6 months notice to the PCO. The experiment with PMS, however, can only be tried once, so it is important to be absolutely certain that the new GMS contract has more to offer financially. Returning to GMS means there can be no future attempts at PMS for your practice unless there is a change in government policy.

Reasons for considering a switch back to GMS include:

- Good performance in quality areas that could be better rewarded financially under GMS.

- Difficulty achieving contract requirements, such as access targets, that might be less punitive under GMS.

- A generous global sum on offer, due to favourable allocation formula weighting.

- The need for premises development.

- Major IT investment needed.

- The security of a nationally negotiated contract.

Switching back should be delayed until the global sum plus the potential quality income exceed the PMS budget. This will undoubtedly be more likely in 2005/6 than in earlier years, due to the planned increase in quality points from £75 to £120 each.

ACCESS

INTRODUCTION

Achieving improved access has always been a desire of this Labour government that has been resisted by the BMA as a contractual requirement of GPs. However, there are now, within the GMS contract, two references to access: in the 50 points granted in the quality framework, and in the directed enhanced services required of all PCOs.

DEFINITION OF ACCESS

According to the detailed guidance on the quality and outcomes framework, the actual requirements for achieving the 50 points are that a patient should be able to have face-to-face contact with any GP within two working days of their request, and to be able to have access to a primary care professional within 24 hours.

This is the definition for England. In Wales, there is only the requirement to see an appropriate professional within 24 hours. In Scotland, there is only the requirement to see a member of the Primary Care Team within 48 hours.

Exceptions to this definition include:

* Situations in which the patient does not wish to be seen within 48 hours.

* Situations wherein the patient specifies a particular professional.

* Requests for emergency or urgent treatment.

* Pre-planned elective treatment or care programmes.

* Out-of-hours coverage.

* Planned closures, e.g. public holidays/staff training.

FINANCES

In 2004/5, the 50 quality points for access will be worth an average of £1250 per GP, rising to £2000 in 2005/6. This is on a par with the number of points for achieving a blood pressure below 150/90 in 70% of all your hypertensives.

The directed enhanced service is priced at £5000 for 2003/4 per 5500 patients. This applies in England and Wales. In Scotland, most practices will continue to be paid via the Scottish Primary Care Collaborative for advanced access, although other methods of meeting the target also qualify.

Half the money for the enhanced service is paid at the beginning of the year, with the balance paid at the end if the target has been achieved.

Approximately 84% of practices in England were already offering appointments within 48 hours, according to a review of the NHS Plan published in March 2003.

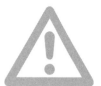

MANAGER'S TIP

Staff commitment to achieving 48-hour access, including bonus systems, can be very useful.

MEETING THE TARGETS FOR ACCESS

ADVANCED ACCESS, BY SIR JOHN OLDHAM

The government has given a high priority to improving access, itself a response to complaint from patients. Within the GMS contract there are two references to access in the 50 points granted in the quality framework, and in the directed enhanced services requested of all PCOs.

In 2004/5 the 50 quality points for access are worth an average of £1250 per GP rising to £2000 in 2005/6. This is on a par with the number of points for achieving a blood pressure below 150/90 in 70% of all your hypotenuses >check figures<. In March 2003 a review of the NHS Plan showed 84% of practices offering appointment within 48 hours.

The National Primary Care Development Team has now worked with over 3500 practices covering 26 million of the population to help them improve access. This has been done through the Primary Care collaborative. The system advocated is advanced access, which helps practices achieve a balance between demand for services and the capacity to deliver them. Many traditional systems work on the basis of "urgent" and routine, with fights, variance and inconsistency over what is or is not urgent. The result is blocking off large numbers of appointments for urgencies. People have to prove they need them, which then transfers demand to subsequent days and builds up a wait or "backlog" of 4, 5, 6 days or whatever. The initiative assumption is that if you improve access and don't keep people waiting you will be flooded out, and people will abuse the access with loads of minor conditions. The reality is different; in fact, patients don't have to "play the system", engineer an urgency or book just in case they need to (Table 3) – they can contrast the different forms of access: traditional, open and advanced.

Traditional access
- Over full appointment schedules
- Work pushed forward from the past to "protect today"
- Urgent/routine appointment types
- Potential long waits for routine appointments
- High DNA rates
- Inequality of access
- Patients "game" the system
- High demand for out-of-hours services
- Backlog of routine work
- Considerable "noise" in the system from patients' complaints
- Stressful environment for practice staff

Open access
- Over full schedules
- Attempts to deal with demand on the day
- Capacity gained by working harder/longer
- Long waits for patients in the surgery
- Urgent/routine split
- Patients game the system to be seen as "urgent"
- Little control over workload
- Considerable "noise" in the system from patients' complaints
- Stressful environment for practice staff

Outcomes of advanced access
- The handling of demand has been altered and face-to-face consultations are used more effectively
- Work pulled into today to "protect the future"
- No distinction between urgent and routine appointments
- Maximum control over workload
- No backlog (capacity and demand are in equilibrium each day)
- DNAs significantly reduced
- Greater equality of access
- No need for patients to "game" the system
- Less "noise" in the system
- Reduced demand for out-of-hours services
- High practice staff and patient satisfaction

Table 3. Characteristics of the various access models (adapted from Murray)

There are five key components to advanced access.

- Understand the demand.

- Shape the handling of demand.

- Match capacity to demand.

- Have contingency plans.

- Communicate the change in advance to patients and staff.

Understand the profile of demand

- Record each day the total appointment requests in a practice (regardless of the day to which the appointment is actually assigned). This should include telephone requests, requests made in person, and follow-ups. Do this for a week. Compare the daily demand with appointments offered.

- Analyse how many appointments (%) each day are follow-ups (e.g. Monday 10%, Tuesday 20%, Wednesday 30%, Thursday 30%, Friday 10%).

The surprising thing is that most times capacity equals demand. It is just 4, 5, 6 days too late. And demand is predictable; one week is pretty much like another, one winter pretty much like the last.

Adjust the handling of demand

Shaping the handling of demand

Exploring different ways to handle demand appropriately means that practices can make the best use of their capacity, and offer patients a choice of ways in which to access care.

'Shaping' in ways such as introducing telephone consultations, telephone management of home visit and same day requests, email for repeat prescription requests and altering the frequency of follow-up appointments creates capacity by reducing the number of face-to-face appointments. Reducing the backlog of long waits means that patients no longer book 'just in case' their condition does not improve and they can't get an appointment, reducing unnecessary consultations and 'Did Not Attends' (DNAs).

'Shaping' the handling of demand often uncovers hidden capacity, which in cases such as Priory Fields Partnership, a 3rd Wave practice in Huntingdonshire, is much needed (Figure 10).

Priory Fields Partnership, Huntingdonshire PCT

When Priory Fields Partnership joined the Collaborative in March 2001, the practice had a 12-day wait for a routine appointment. The first step for GP Andrew Wright and Nurse Sophie Kellen was to measure demand; their analysis showed that the practice was at least 170 appointments short each week. Realising that more could be done with their existing capacity, PDSAs were developed to test out telephone consultations, develop nurse triage and review follow-up practices.

During the course of the Collaborative, the practice ran into a crisis: two part-time GPs left. Despite this, the practice continued improving access, clearing the backlog of appointments and introducing advanced access at the start of October 2001.

The changes introduced by the practice team have freed up hidden capacity: nurse triage has reduced GP face-to-face consultations by 45%, home visits have reduced by 25%, follow-ups have reduced from 47% to 35%. 99% of patients are able to get an appointment on their day of choice, 95% with their GP of choice.

One patient wrote to congratulate the team:

'Whenever I phone the surgery or come in, the reception staff are extremely friendly, helpful and most importantly smile! It is now a pleasure to come into the surgery and I would like to congratulate you and your staff for the massive improvements that have taken place'.

Advanced access has also provided the practice with a new approach to recruitment. Based on their new knowledge of demand, the team has developed a precise picture of how much more clinical time is needed to offer patients a high quality service and clinicians a safe, sustainable working environment. A GP from a local practice has been recruited to provide one session of diabetic support and so free up doctor time and a GP has been recruited at eight sessions rather than six to give the team some extra capacity.

Nurse 'triage' of same day demand has become a commonly tested approach to managing demand and ensuring that patients see an appropriate member of the primary health care team. Rather than the traditional concept of triage as a means of defining urgency, triage is used as a way of managing each patient's needs. Whether by telephone or face-to-face, the interaction is designed to either address the problem there and then or to assess which member of the team the patient should see.

An increasingly important aspect of shaping demand is increasing self-help. Many do this for minor illness using ideas such as a patient-manned desk with advice leaflets or video library, a consistent line on managing minor illnesses. Key is moulding advice material to what patients tell you they need, rather than the other way round. However, the big gains are to be made by involving those with enduring illness in the management of their care. Evidence demonstrates not only an improvement in the clincial outcome, but also reduced consultation rate.

Match capacity to demand

Reduce the backlog of appointments. Having changed the demand the next step is to balance the appointment capacity with that demand by ensuring the daily appointment profile matches the demand profile that has been worked out. When moving to this new system there will still be an overhang from the old system of people waiting to be seen: "the backlog".

We are going to recommend a sequencing of events that people experience shows reduces the backlog of appointments.

1. We define backlog as the number of days between today and the earliest availability of an appointment

2. A useful measure of the backlog (which helps to smooth out large day-to-day fluctuations) is the time a patient would have to wait to access the third available appointment slot at the time of making the request. Although this sounds clumsy, it proves very useful information for planning, e.g. if the third available appointment with a doctor or nurse is in X days, and there are normally Y appointments per day, then the backlog $Z = X - Y$. This means that Z appointments need to be "worked through" before the backlog will be cleared.

3. Set up some simple systems for alternative access and a contingency policy (i.e. what happens automatically if someone is off sick or on holiday, or during an epidemic).

4. Match the capacity of the appointment system to predicted daily demand.

5. Set a date by which the backlog will be cleared. This will require hard work and need short-term additional capacity, e.g. additional time each surgery or alternative shift patterns. Once a stable state is reached, i.e. daily capacity = demand, then it becomes easier to manage daily any day-to-day variations in the predicted demand for appointments.

Matching capacity to reshaped demand

As well as looking at simple ways to shift capacity to where it is needed, many practices have looked at developing the capacity within their teams. Optimising how people are working, or developing new skills, can lead to dramatic improvements in access.

Developing skills within the practice team frees up GP and nurse appointments to manage patients in the most appropriate way. As well as shaping demand with telephone and email consultations, 1st Wave Bridge House Surgery in Stratford PCT has introduced a health care assistant, trained reception staff to undertake BP checks, phlebotomy and new patient registrations and introduced nurse-led clinics and new follow-up procedures for HRT, COCP and BP checks. Their GP 3rd available appointment has reduced from 12 days to 1, and the improvement maintained.

Frances Street Surgery in Doncaster PCT has used the advanced access model and their PMS pilot status to develop a nurse-led primary care service. Understanding demand enabled the practice to reduce its waiting times, freeing up capacity to expand nurse work further. The practice has a triage service, minor illness clinics, heart care and hypertension clinics, all of which are nurse-led. Many of the services involve the wider nurse team – District Nurses, Health Visitors and Community Nurses. Nurses handle up to 80% of the practice's demand, and GPs have been able to extend the length of their appointments without working longer hours. The practice has also piloted a patient advice service jointly with the local council. The advice worker can provide personal support to patients on a wide range of non-medical issues. An evaluation based on a group of patients before and after using the service has shown a 30% reduction in GP consultations.

Contingency Plans

Sustaining improvements in access

Practices that have implemented advanced access have demonstrated that the system is sustainable but that this can only be achieved by proactive, ongoing management. The key is in recognising that advanced access is not an endpoint but a dynamic process.

Having practical contingency plans means that a practice can manage at times when capacity will be reduced, whether expectedly due to holiday or unexpectedly due to sickness or increased demand. Such times can often mean increased workload for a short time, but it means that delays do not build up again, the system will return to normal once full capacity returns.

Yarm Medical Practice Contingency Plans		F/T	P/T
1	If one GP away for a full week then no change with appointments		
2a	If one GP + Nurse Practitioner away for full week – extra appointments to be put in by remaining GPs over the week:	8	6
2b	Drop Administration Session		
2c	Nurse triage to continue, but to be the responsibility of the Practice Nurse covering the Treatment Room	8	6
3a	If two GPs away for a full week – extra appointments to be put in by remaining GPs over the week:		
3b	If needed, Nurse Practitioner to swap her Treatment Session for a bookable Nurse Practitioner session. Other practice nurses asked to cover treatment room as part of their flexible contract		
3c	Drop Administration Session		
3d	Cancel Practice Meeting – then no change with appointments		
4a	If Nurse Practitioner away – then no change with appointments		
4b	Nurse triage to continue but to be the responsibility of the Practice Nurse covering the Treatment Room		

Popular contingencies include increasing the amount of 'shaping' carried out, particularly the telephone management, and postponing meetings and outside commitments until capacity is restored to the necessary levels.

Sunnybank Medical Centre is a 1st Wave practice with 9400 patients in Bradford South and West PCT. The practice joined the Collaborative with a third available appointment of 9 days for GPs, and around 160-200 DNAs each month. Their initial measurement of demand showed a shortfall of 20-30% of appointments. After measuring demand, the practice team has used PDSAs to introduce changes including telephone consultations, group consultations, skill mixing including introducing a Health Care Assistant and Treatment Room nurse and extending the role of the reception team to include phlebotomy. Due to their understanding of demand, the practice has been able to contract long-term locum cover as part of their contingency plans. The third available appointment is 0 days for GPs and 1 day for nurses at June 2002, 18 months after introducing the change. DNAs are now typically less than 40 per month, around 1% of appointments.

South Norwood Hill Medical Centre in 1st Wave North Croydon PCT implemented advanced access in July 2000, the first practice on the Collaborative to do so. They have measured demand and capacity since then and, using process control methods, are able to demonstrate that their system remains stable after two years. Their contingency plans include flexing the length of surgeries and converting clinics to routine appointments when GPs are away. The practice has experienced a reduction in DNAs from 12% of appointments to 5%. Demand for out of hours services has also fallen and they have not needed locum cover since they introduced the system.

Communication

It is important to have a definitive plan for communication both with staff and patients before AA day. For staff they need to understand the difference and the script – *most crucially, that pre-bookable appointments are part of advanced access*. When the demand and number of follow-ups are established in understanding demand, you should have allocated a proportion of the appointments to pre-bookable according to the maths. This will need to be adjusted over the first month with experience. Responses from receptionists to "ring on the day" to avoid pre-booking are unhelpful and an irritant. Secondly, communication with patients needs to be deliberately high profile and continued for nearly a year. People attend infrequently and if they don't know there is a new system they will behave as per the old system.

Debunking the myths

Finally, let us debunk the myths surrounding improving access (Table 4).

Myth 1	Improving access increases demand. No – practices show plateauing or decrease, and certainly a decrease in visits.
Myth 2	Improving access is about speeding people through to the detriment of quality. No – the practices on the Collaborative substantially improved outcomes for coronary heart disease as well as improving access. Many managed to lengthen consultation time.
Myth 3	Advanced access is only concerned with seeing people on the day they ring. No – advanced access is about seeing people when they need to be seen, including the ability to book in advance.

Table 4. Myths surrounding improving access

Further information is available at www.npdt.org or your local NPDT Centre.

ALTERNATIVES TO ADVANCED ACCESS

Open access, whereby patients turn up at the surgery between set times without an appointment, is, perhaps, the traditional model of running general practice. The advantages are:

- Access targets are met.

- There is no friction between reception and patients.

- Patients are seen on the day of their choice, no matter how urgent.

Some of the problems with this method are:

- Patients dictate workload spread.

- There are long waits in the waiting room.

- Surgery is of unpredictable duration.

A hybrid system, whereby most patients pre-book but extras are seen on the same day, is currently the most popular method of running general practice in the UK.

Under this system the access targets can be met by a combination of same-day appointments and a sliding scale of thresholds for releasing appointments in advance. Predicting the pattern of demand is crucial to success. So having more appointments free on a Monday, for example, is essential, as that is the day of highest demand for same-day appointments.

To provide same-day appointments without increasing overall workload means blocking off those appointments, and releasing them to patients on the day they are needed. A few appointments will need to be bookable two working days in advance in order to meet the access targets. The remainder can be booked in advance for routine follow-ups and to accommodate those patients who organise themselves a week or two ahead.

MONITORING

Having a dedicated member of staff to monitor availability of appointments is essential. On occasions of higher-than-expected demand, extra appointments need to be accommodated by surgeries at short notice. This need not mean extra work for the doctors, but can be achieved by altering the booking category of one or two appointment slots (changing them from, say, a book-on-the-day to a 48-hour access).

Gaming the system in this way can help to achieve 48-hour access without creating extra work for the doctors of the practice.

TROUBLESHOOTING

If achieving the access targets seems impossible, then one has to ask whether the practice is providing enough medical/nursing appointments to meet demand. So long as you are confident that the system cannot be managed more efficiently, or even manipulated cynically for the sake of qualifying for target payments, then extra time will be needed.

This does not, however, mean that the partners will have to extend their consulting later into the evenings. Access targets can be met by:

- Shifting work between doctors/nurses.

- Employing salaried medical staff.

- Reducing demand by telephone triage.

- Improving access to telephone advice.

- Contracting out to neighbouring providers.

But remember that whenever changes are made to free up 48-hour appointments, those appointments must be protected for just such use. There's no point shifting all your contraception work to the practice nurse just so you've got more time to see the extras on the same day.

Access appointments should be colour-coded on the receptionist's appointment screen, and released to the public at exactly the right time so as to qualify for the target payments.

SENIORITY

Seniority payments under the new GMS contract reward length of service in the NHS. From 2003/4 they will start to be awarded to GMS principals with at least 9 years service, and will include all superannuable years, whether in hospital, or as a GP registrar, salaried GP or partner.

The payments are not the so-called wisdom and experience payments that were mentioned in the contract framework document, published by the BMA in April 2002. How, indeed, would one reward wisdom? Just picture the scene. "Oh wise and enlightened senior partner, what shall we do about this prescribing overspend? Give us your answer and you win £6k."

Seniority was, and remains, a loyalty payment.

The pricing structure has been fixed so that, in theory, no one is worse off than they were under the previous seniority rules. For example, the GP with 6 years' service as a principal (i.e. in receipt of Basic Practice Allowance) who has just started to receive the first seniority payment (£600 for 2002/3), is also likely to have at least 1 year's experience as a GP registrar, 2 as a senior house officer and 1 as a pre-registration house officer. Thus, 10 years' service under the NHS equates to £612 seniority in 2003/4, a pay rise of £12.

Unlike the Red Book, the new GMS contract rewards every extra year's service with a higher seniority payment, rather than the four major steps at 6, 13, 19 and 25 years. So, the GP in the above example will receive £729 in 2004/5 and £1184 in 2005/6. GPs who spent longer than the minimum number of years in training, and those who have worked in other fields of NHS medicine, can add up all their years' service and arrive at a higher seniority payment.

The maximum payment available in the year 2003/4 will be £10,317 for a GP with 47 years' service in the NHS. This GP would be at least 70 years old. The 60-year-old GP who has spent his or her entire working life in the NHS without a break could amass 37 years' seniority or £9157 in 2003/4. This figure will rise by just under £2000 over the following 2 years. These figures are all greater than the Red Book payment of £8225, the maximum seniority pay available in the year 2002/3. They are, however, lower than the total seniority plus the £2000 a year "golden handcuffs" payment that is missing from the new contract.

Seniority payments only reward length of NHS service. GPs who qualified in the UK and then spent time working abroad may find their seniority pay reduced under the new GMS contract.

Under the Red Book, most practices awarded seniority payments to the partner who "earned" them. The income was treated as a prior share in the practice accounts and as a small financial reward for length of service.

Now that the seniority figures are potentially greater, they could be used to award senior members of the partnership with time away from the practice. In this case, seniority would be paid to the practice and used towards funding salaried GP time.

A sum of £7000 a year, for example, would pay for a salaried doctor to do one session a week, thus freeing up a partner for the same amount of time. As doctors approach retirement age, some would rather reduce their practice commitment than receive extra income, and the new seniority scales make this possible. In fact, £7000 seniority can be reached by the age of 50 with uninterrupted NHS service to 2003/4.

An agreement to pay seniority into the practice could result in a net profit to the practice, even after paying for salaried time. This profit is, of course, shared by all the partners, including the seniors.

Deciding how to treat seniority payments within the practice should be discussed with the advice of the practice accountant. The final decision should be spelt out clearly in the partnership agreement to avoid misunderstanding.

APPENDIX 1:
COMPUTER RESOURCES

The financial aspects of the new GMS contract can be enhanced by successful use of the practice's computer system. Two areas of computer use are most relevant: data entry and audit.

If data are entered into the computer in the correct way, particularly for chronic disease management, then it is easier to prove that Quality and Outcome targets have been reached. By auditing these data in the right way, the process of data retrieval is simplified, and the whole task of submitting the annual verification report to the PCO is made less painful.

The three main computer software suppliers in general practice – EMIS, Torex and InPractice Systems – all use similar methods of data recording. Essentially, this is in the form of a structured data grid that can be called up on-screen during the consultation and will prompt the user to enter predefined data in sequence. The grids can either be customised by the user, or patched in as a download from the company.

EMIS

Tel.: 08701 205527 Sales & Marketing
Tel.: 0870 1221177 Field Operations Team
Tel.: 0870 1221133 General support
www.emis-online.com

Refer to the manual or contact the trainers in the Field Operations Team for detailed guidance on use of the Graphical Template Editor.

Log on to the on-line common room using your EMIS customer number.

New contract templates will be provided either as downloads from the website, or as patches available on request via the NHS Net or direct to the practice by ISDN line.

Torex

Tel.: 01295 274200 Reception
Tel.: 0870 6095533 Sales
www.torex.com

Torex's system, Premier Synergy, uses SOPHIE (Screening Patient Health in an Interactive Environment). There are standard SOPHIEs which can be customised using the Graphical SOPHIE Editor.

Log in to Torex using your user name and password to download SOPHIEs from Torex. These are also transferable from PCOs and other practices' systems.

Data extraction is possible with MIQUEST or customised searches can be designed.

Contact Torex to arrange for a trainer to visit the practice for advice on using the Graphical SOPHIE Editor, or refer to the manual.

InPractice Systems

Tel.: 020 75017000 Head Office
Tel.: 024 76422334 Training
www.inps.co.uk

InPractice Systems' primary care software, known as Vision, uses Structured Data Areas (or grids) which can be custom built and embedded in the consultation manager screen for use during the consultation. There are several already on the system, but they are not specific to the new contract and need customising.

To learn how to do this, either consult the manual or call the above number to arrange for a trainer to visit the practice.

On the INPS website there is a free download for auditing the Q&O data for the new GMS contract. This feeds the data into Excel for printing off and submitting to the PCO for verification and payment.

APPENDIX 2: SAMPLE MEDICO-LEGAL REPORT

(LORD WOOLF'S REQUIREMENTS IN ITALICS)

MEDICAL REPORT

on

Mr H

DOB

Address

****

Date of Accident – 14th October 2002

Solicitors Reference

?????????

****

Date 15th January 2003

Interview Faringdon Health Centre

3.15 pm 15th January 2003

"I understand that my duty in writing this report is to help the court on the matters within my expertise. I understand that this duty overrides any obligation to the person from whom I have received instructions or by whom I am being paid.

I confirm that I have complied with that duty in writing my report."

Dr Simon Richard Cartwright

MB BS MRCGP

General Medical Practitioner

The Accident

Mr H was involved in a road traffic accident on 14th October 2002. He was driving a stationary car, which was hit from behind by another car. At the moment of impact Mr H was wearing the driver's seat belt. The car was fitted with a headrest.

Injuries Sustained

As a result of the road traffic accident on14th October 2002, Mr H sustained the following injuries.

1. Acute psychological shock in the form of agitation, and anxiety.

2. A flexion extension injury to the cervical spine in the form of a typical whiplash injury.

3. Lower back and groin pain.

4. Right wrist pain.

Treatment

Mr H saw a locum GP the day after the accident and was advised to take Voltarol and co-codamol for pain relief. He was changed to Neurofen and paracetamol due to diarrhoea. He took the tablets for a total of 3 to 4 weeks.

He has had a series of six sessions with an osteopath for the treatment of neck and back pain as well.

Chronological Progression of Psychological Symptoms

The acute psychological shock suffered by Mr H persisted for approximately 10 minutes. On the second day after the accident he noticed that he had developed a generalised anxiety. He became depressed and irritable due to persistent pain, causing inability to have sex and to sleep well. This persisted for about a month and was thereafter better.

Chronological Progression of Physical Symptoms

The whiplash injury caused pain in the neck which persisted for 2 weeks and was then replaced by a burning sensation in the neck and right wrist. This was thereafter exacerbated by prolonged use of the right arm, for example when driving or typing.

The lower back and groin pains developed immediately and persisted for about 4 weeks, settling down after treatment by the osteopath.

Present Situation

The present situation is that Mr H continues to be troubled by burning in the cervical spine and right wrist on prolonged use of the right arm.

He has no persistence of the anxiety-related problems from the accident.

Loss Consequential to Injury

As a result of the road traffic accident on 14th October 2002, Mr H was unable to work for 3 weeks. He also found that, because of persistent neck pain and lower back pain, he could not drive for about a month, he could not go beating for the local shoot for a month and could do no gardening for 6 weeks. He was unable to do any DIY for 6 weeks. He has not been able to ride a horse since the accident, partly due to symptoms, and partly due to worry that he may exacerbate the symptoms again.

On Examination

Mr H is a healthy-looking 45-year-old man with a normal posture and gait.

1. <u>Cervical Spine</u>
   There is no abnormality of posture of the cervical spine. There is a full range of normal movement in all directions, both active and passive. There is no tenderness of the cervical spine nor of the trapezii bilaterally.

2. <u>Thoracic Spine</u>
There is no abnormality of the thoracic curvature. Mr H is non-tender over the spinous processes. He has a good range of movement of the thoracic spine, both active and passive in all directions.

3. <u>Lumbar Spine</u>
There is no abnormality of the lumbar lordosis. He has a good range of movement in all directions. There is no tenderness in the lumbar region on palpation of the bony spine and the paraspinal muscles.

4. <u>Upper Limbs</u>
Mr H has full range of movement at the shoulders, elbows and wrists with normal upper limb neurology. There is no objective sign of weakness and sensation is normal. There is no sign of bruising or tenderness. The right wrist appears normal.

5. <u>Lower Limbs</u>
There is a full range of movement in all joints. Lower limb neurology is normal.

6. <u>Chest</u>
There are no abnormal markings of the chest. There is no tenderness over either clavicle or of any of the ribs or sternum. The lung fields are clear.

Past Medical History

Mr H reported an episode of temporary low back pain 10 years ago, requiring treatment from an osteopath. He denied any neck problems, but referral to his medical records revealed an episode of neck pain in 1996, requiring physiotherapy, and another episode in 1997 requiring physiotherapy.

Summary

Mr H was involved in a road traffic accident on 14th October 2002 in which his car was struck by another car. His injuries consisted of acute psychological stress, whiplash, lower back and groin pain, and right wrist pain. His persisting symptoms include neck and right wrist burning on prolonged use of the right arm.

It is important to note that I have had access to his medical records in compiling this report. Mr H appears to be a reliable witness and his injuries are consistent with the reported accident.

Prospects on Open Job Market

At the present time Mr H has returned to his previous job as a surveyor. There is no reason to suspect that his prospects in the open job market will be in any way compromised by the accident.

Reasonableness

It is my opinion that the amount of time taken off work as a result of the accident was reasonable.

Recommendations

Mr H's neck and wrist burning persists to this date. I would anticipate gradual resolution of this problem over the next 3 to 6 months. If his symptoms have not resolved in that time I would recommend further examination by an Orthopaedic Surgeon.

I believe that the facts I have stated in this report are true and that the opinions I have expressed are correct.

Dr S. R. CARTWRIGHT, MBBS MRCGP DCH DRCOG

APPENDIX 3: VASECTOMY CLINIC PAPERWORK

Private and Confidential

Mr M M
10 Church Lane
Clanfield
Oxon
OX18 2BA

Dear Mr M

I now have the results of both your semen specimens, which are all clear.

I confirm that your vasectomy is now a reliable method of contraception and that other methods can be abandoned.

Best wishes

Yours sincerely

Dr Simon Cartwright

<u>INSTRUCTIONS FOR COLLECTING</u>

<u>**SEMINAL SPECIMENS**</u>

1. A specimen of semen is required 4 months after the operation, and a further specimen 2 weeks later.

2. The specimen must be collected in the morning. It is best to leave a few nights without intercourse beforehand.

   It must be passed directly into the jar provided. It may be collected either by incomplete intercourse and withdrawal, or by hand, but a sheath must not be used. The whole of the specimen is required.

3. After collecting, replace the screw cap, making sure that it is very tight. Remember to write the date on the jar and the form. Put the jar in the bag attached to the back of the form, remove the adhesive cover-strip and fold the top of the bag over. Hand in the specimen at your surgery before 10 am Monday to Friday.

4. When the results of two specimens have been received, the Coxwell Clinic will inform you of the result in writing.

<u>NOTES FOR YOUR GUIDANCE AFTER YOUR</u>

<u>VASECTOMY OPERATION</u>

When you leave the clinic you should go straight home and spend the next 2 days quietly resting. This is to avoid the risk of bleeding, which might be caused by disturbance of the operation site. It is often the people who think they are fit for shopping, gardening or squash who subsequently have post-operative problems.

You should avoid alcohol for 24 hours as this also tends to cause bleeding.

It is sensible to take a painkiller such as aspirin or paracetamol before the anaesthetic wears off after about an hour.

The stitches should not need attention: they dissolve and fall out after about 10 days.

Change the dressing daily until the wound has healed. Do not soak the area before healing has occurred: make do with a shower or splash wash.

You may resume sporting activities and sexual intercourse after 10 days. If your job involves much heavy activity, it may be wise to have 3 or 4 days off work.

Some tenderness, bruising and swelling is to be expected. More severe bruising and swelling affects about one in 50 patients. If you are worried by what you think are unusually severe problems, phone the clinic for advice on the number below.

Do not forget to continue alternative contraceptive precautions until you know that you have had two consecutive negative semen counts.

The longer you can postpone submitting the semen specimens for testing, the more likely they are to be clear; by being patient you may avoid the need to repeat the tests. Wait for at least 4 months.

Private and Confidential

Mr M M
10 Church Lane
Clanfield
Oxon
OX18 2BA

Dear Mr M

The appointment for your vasectomy is: Friday 6.11.2003 at 1.30 p.m.

On the day of the operation you will be examined and, if considered suitable, be given the operation under local anaesthetic.

For this we charge a registration fee of £90, payable when the appointment is confirmed, and £50 at the time of the operation (cash or cheque made payable to Dr S. Cartwright).

To confirm that you will be attending, please send the £90 registration fee to the address below with the signed consent form from your doctor.

Before you come for the operation **please shave the whole scrotum**. Please bring with you a pair of tight pants. After the operation, which takes about 35 minutes, you will not need to stay longer than a short time to rest, but it would be wise to spend the next 2 days quietly at home. Keep the small wound covered and don't get it wet. There will be no stitches needing removal.

Four months after the operation you should submit a specimen of semen for examination and a second specimen 2 weeks later. Specimen jars will be provided at the time of the operation and these can be handed in to your surgery for transport to the hospital. **Until two negative tests have been secured you should take extra contraceptive precautions**. You will be advised of the result in writing.

If you have any questions about the operation, please telephone me, Dr Simon Cartwright, on the number below.

Yours sincerely

Dr Simon Cartwright

6.11.2003

Dr Tony Copperfield
The Surgery
High Street
Essex CN12 4DX

Dear

Re: Mr M M, 10 Church Lane, Clanfield Oxon, OX18 2BA. Tel.:

Thank you for your referral of 12.10.2003.

We have undertaken his vasectomy today, 6.11.2003.

He should rest after the operation and he would be wise to take the next 2 days off work. The small wound should be kept covered and not wetted. There will be no stitches needing removal.

The patient has been given two jars and path forms to submit a specimen 4 months after the operation and a second sample 2 weeks later. When two consecutive negatives have been reported we will send him confirmation in writing. Two specimens without a single sperm are needed. This still leaves a risk of spontaneous reversal of one in five thousand.

We would be grateful if the specimens could be collected by the laboratory transport system from your surgery. You will not receive an invoice from the laboratory.

If any post-operative problems arise please don't hesitate to contact me on the number below.

Best wishes

Yours sincerely

Dr Simon Cartwright

Date applied	Date of operation	Name: M M
		Address: 10 Church Lane
		Clanfield
		Oxon
		OX18 2BA

Deposit:	Date:	Tel. Home:
		Tel. Work:
Balance:	Date:	Number:

Referring GP:	
Dr Tony Copperfield	Nurse informed
The Surgery	
High Street	
Essex	
CN12 4DX	

Age: Partner's age:

Children:

Counselling: Irreversible: Consent form:
                              Delayed effect:
                              Side-effects:

Previous surgery: Bleeding tendency: Heart Disease:

Medication: Reactions to LA: Miscellaneous:

Operation: **Date:**

LA 2% Lignocaine with adrenaline:

Surgeon: Dr S. Cartwright

Nurse:

Technique:

Post Op:

Semenalysis results:

Clearance given:

APPENDIX 4: PATIENTS' SATISFACTION QUESTIONNAIRES

GPAQ

GPAQ is a patient questionnaire that has been developed at the National Primary Care Research and Development Centre in Manchester for the 2003 GP contract. Building on several years of development and testing, GPAQ helps practices find out what patients think about their care. It specifically focuses on aspects of general practice that are not covered elsewhere in the Quality and Outcomes Framework – for example, access, inter-personal aspects of care and continuity of care.

Practice [ ][ ][ ]   Patient [ ][ ][ ]

The General Practice Assessment Questionnaire (GPAQ)

Dear Patient

We would be grateful if you would complete this survey about your general practice.

Your practice wants to provide the highest standard of care. Feedback from this survey will enable the practice to identify areas that may need improvement. Your opinions are therefore very valuable.

Please answer ALL the questions that apply to you. There are no right or wrong answers and staff will NOT be able to identify your individual responses.

Thank you.

		None	Once or twice	Three or four times	Five or six times	Seven times or more
1	In the past 12 months, **how many times** have you seen a doctor from your practice?	☐ 1	☐ 2	☐ 3	☐ 4	☐ 5

		Very poor	Poor	Fair	Good	Very good	Excellent
2	How do you rate the way you are treated by **receptionists** at your practice?	☐ 1	☐ 2	☐ 3	☐ 4	☐ 5	☐ 6

		Very poor	Poor	Fair	Good	Very good	Excellent
3	a) How do you rate the **hours** that your practice is open for appointments?	☐ 1	☐ 2	☐ 3	☐ 4	☐ 5	☐ 6

		Early morning	Lunch times	Evenings	Weekends	None, I am satisfied
	b) What **additional** hours would you like the practice to be open? (please tick all that apply)	☐ 1	☐ 2	☐ 3	☐ 4	☐ 5

4 Thinking of times when you want to see a **particular** doctor (please tick one box only):

	Same day	Next working day	Within 2 working days	Within 3 working days	Within 4 working days	5 or more working days	Does not apply
a) How **quickly** do you usually get to see that doctor?	☐ 1	☐ 2	☐ 3	☐ 4	☐ 5	☐ 6	☐ 7

	Very poor	Poor	Fair	Good	Very good	Excellent	Does not apply
b) How do you rate this?	☐ 1	☐ 2	☐ 3	☐ 4	☐ 5	☐ 6	☐ 7

© GPAQ is copyright of the National Primary Care Research and Development Centre, University of Manchester and Safran/NEMCH

www.gpaq.info

Postal Version 1.0

5 Thinking of times when you are willing to see **any** doctor (please tick one box only):

	Same day	Next working day	Within 2 working days	Within 3 working days	Within 4 working days	5 or more working days	Does not apply
a) How **quickly** do you usually get seen?	☐1	☐2	☐3	☐4	☐5	☐6	☐7
	Very poor	Poor	Fair	Good	Very good	Excellent	Does not apply
b) How do you rate this?	☐1	☐2	☐3	☐4	☐5	☐6	☐7

	Yes	No	Don't know/never needed to
6 If you need to see a GP **urgently**, can you normally get seen on the same day?	☐1	☐2	☐3

	5 minutes or less	6–10 minutes	11–20 minutes	21–30 minutes	More than 30 minutes
7 a) How long do you usually have to **wait** at the practice for your consultations to begin? (please tick one box only)	☐1	☐2	☐3	☐4	☐5
	Very poor	Poor	Fair	Good	Very good	Excellent
b) How do you rate this?	☐1	☐2	☐3	☐4	☐5	☐6

8 Thinking of times you have **phoned** the practice, how do you rate the following?

	Very poor	Poor	Fair	Good	Very good	Excellent	Don't know/ never tried
a) Ability **to get through to** the practice on the phone?	☐1	☐2	☐3	☐4	☐5	☐6	☐7
b) Ability to **speak to** a doctor on the phone when you have a question or need medical advice?	☐1	☐2	☐3	☐4	☐5	☐6	☐7

The next questions ask about your <u>usual doctor.</u> If you don't have a 'usual doctor', answer about the one doctor at your practice whom you know best. If you don't know any of the doctors, go straight to question 11.

	Always	Almost always	A lot of the time	Some of the time	Almost never	Never
9 a) In general, how often do you see your **usual doctor**?	☐1	☐2	☐3	☐4	☐5	☐6
	Very poor	Poor	Fair	Good	Very good	Excellent
b) How do you rate this?	☐1	☐2	☐3	☐4	☐5	☐6

10 Thinking about **when you consult** your usual doctor, how do you rate the following?

	Very poor	Poor	Fair	Good	Very good	Excellent	Does not apply
a) How **thoroughly** the doctor asks about your symptoms and how you are feeling	☐1	☐2	☐3	☐4	☐5	☐6	☐7
b) How well the doctor **listens** to what you have to say	☐1	☐2	☐3	☐4	☐5	☐6	☐7
c) How well the doctor **puts you at ease** during your physical examination	☐1	☐2	☐3	☐4	☐5	☐6	☐7
d) How much the doctor **involves you in decisions** about your care	☐1	☐2	☐3	☐4	☐5	☐6	☐7
e) How well the doctor **explains** your problems or any treatment that you need	☐1	☐2	☐3	☐4	☐5	☐6	☐7
f) The amount of **time** your doctor spends with you	☐1	☐2	☐3	☐4	☐5	☐6	☐7
g) The doctor's **patience** with your questions or worries	☐1	☐2	☐3	☐4	☐5	☐6	☐7
h) The doctor's **caring and concern** for you	☐1	☐2	☐3	☐4	☐5	☐6	☐7

11 Have you seen a **nurse** from your practice in the past 12 months   ☐1 Yes – go to question 12   ☐2 No – go to question 13

12 Thinking about the **nurse(s) you have seen,** how do you rate the following?

	Very poor	Poor	Fair	Good	Very good	Excellent
a) How well they **listen** to what you say	☐1	☐2	☐3	☐4	☐5	☐6
b) The **quality** of care they provide	☐1	☐2	☐3	☐4	☐5	☐6
c) How well they **explain** your health problems or any treatment that you need	☐1	☐2	☐3	☐4	☐5	☐6

13 All things considered, how **satisfied** are you with your practice? (please tick only one box)

☐1 Completely satisfied   ☐2 Very satisfied   ☐3 Fairly satisfied   ☐4 Neutral

☐5 Fairly dissatisfied   ☐6 Very dissatisfied   ☐7 Completely dissatisfied

Finally, it will help us to understand your answers if you could tell us a little about yourself:

14 Are you:

☐ 1 Male   ☐ 2 Female

15 How old are you? _____ years

16 Do you have any **long-standing illness, disability or infirmity**? By long-standing we mean anything that has troubled you over a period of time or that is likely to affect you over a period of time

☐ 1 Yes   ☐ 2 No

17 Which **ethnic group** do you belong to? (please tick one box)

☐ 1 White   ☐ 4 Mixed

☐ 2 Black or Black British   ☐ 5 Chinese

☐ 3 Asian or Asian British   ☐ 6 Other ethnic group

18 Is your **accommodation**: (please tick one box)

☐ 1 Owner-occupied/mortgaged?   ☐ 2 Rented or other arrangements?

19 Which of the following best describes you? (please tick one box)

☐ 1 Employed (full or part time, including self-employed)   ☐ 5 Looking after your home/family

☐ 2 Unemployed and looking for work   ☐ 6 Retired from paid work

☐ 3 At school or in full time education   ☐ 7 Other (please describe)................................

☐ 4 Unable to work due to long term sickness   ....

20 We are interested in any other comments you may have. Please write them here.

Is there anything particularly good about your health care?

Is there anything that could be improved?

Any other comments?

Thank you for taking time to complete this questionnaire.

IPQ

In primary care, Client-Focused Evaluations Program (CFEP; http://latis.ex.ac.uk/cfep/) has developed the Improving Practice Questionnaire (IPQ), which is one of the questionnaires approved for use in the Quality and Outcomes framework of the new GP Contract. The questionnaire is structured around commonly agreed standards for general practice (as determined by Royal Colleges of General Practice). The IPQ was informed by Dr John Ware (USA), who was one of the lead authors on patient questionnaires developed by RAND for the Medical Outcomes Study. The IPQ was further refined after extensive consultations with patients, Clinical Governance Leads, other primary care staff and the GP contract negotiators (NHS Confederation and the General Practice Committee of the British Medical Association).

CFEP©   NO.

IMPROVING PRACTICE QUESTIONNAIRE

DOCTOR'S NAME:

YOU CAN HELP THIS GENERAL PRACTICE IMPROVE ITS SERVICE

. The practice and the doctors at this surgery would welcome your honest feedback.

. Please do not write your name on this survey.

. Please read and complete this survey after you have seen the doctor.

PLEASE RATE EACH OF THE FOLLOWING AREAS BY CIRCLING ONE NUMBER ON EACH LINE.

	Poor	Fair	Good	Very Good	Excellent
ABOUT THE PRACTICE					
1. Your level of satisfaction with the practice's opening hours	1	2	3	4	5
2. Ease of contacting the practice on the telephone	1	2	3	4	5
3. Satisfaction with the day and time arranged for your appointment	1	2	3	4	5
4. Chances of seeing a doctor within 48 hours	1	2	3	4	5
5. Opportunity of speaking to a doctor on the telephone when necessary	1	2	3	4	5
6. Comfort level of waiting room (eg. chairs, magazines)	1	2	3	4	5
7. Respect shown for your privacy and confidentiality	1	2	3	4	5
8. Length of time waiting in the practice to see the doctor	1	2	3	4	5
ABOUT THE DOCTOR (*whom you just saw*)					
9. My overall satisfaction with this visit to the doctor is	1	2	3	4	5
10. The warmth of the doctor's greeting to me was	1	2	3	4	5
11. On this visit I would rate the doctor's ability to really listen to me as	1	2	3	4	5
12. The doctor's explanations of things to me were	1	2	3	4	5
13. The extent to which I felt reassured by this doctor was	1	2	3	4	5
14. My confidence in this doctor's ability is	1	2	3	4	5
15. The opportunity the doctor gave me to express my concerns or fears was	1	2	3	4	5
16. The respect shown to me by this doctor was	1	2	3	4	5

PLEASE TURN OVER

SAMPLE ONLY – NOT TO BE COPIED

ABOUT THE DOCTOR (Continued....)	Poor	Fair	Good	Very Good	Excellent
17. The amount of time given to me for this visit was	1	2	3	4	5
18. This doctor's consideration of my personal situation in deciding a treatment or advising me was	1	2	3	4	5
19. The doctor's concern for me as a person in this visit was	1	2	3	4	5
20. The recommendation I would give to my friends about this doctor would be	1	2	3	4	5
ABOUT THE STAFF					
21. The manner in which you are treated by the reception staff	1	2	3	4	5
22. Information provided by the practice about its services (e.g repeat prescriptions, test results, cost of private certificates)	1	2	3	4	5
23. The opportunity for making compliments or complaints to this practice about its service and quality of care	1	2	3	4	5
FINALLY					
24. The information provided by this practice about how to prevent illness and stay healthy (e.g. alcohol use, health risks of smoking, diet habits, etc) was	1	2	3	4	5
25. The availability and administration of reminder systems for ongoing health checks is	1	2	3	4	5
26. The practice's respect of your right to seek a second opinion was....	1	2	3	4	5
27. My overall satisfaction with this general practice	1	2	3	4	5

Any comments about how this <u>practice</u> could improve their service?_____
_____
_____

Any comments about how the <u>doctor</u> could improve?_____
_____
_____

The following questions provide us only with general information about the range of people who have responded to this survey. This information will <u>not</u> be used to identify you and will remain confidential.

How old are you, in years? _____   What is your postcode? _____

Are you ☐ Female   Was this visit with your usual GP?   ☐ Yes

☐ Male   ☐ No

How many years have you been attending this Practice?   ☐ Less than five years

☐ Five to ten years

☐ More than ten years

THANK YOU FOR YOUR TIME AND ASSISTANCE

INDEX

Notes
To save space, the following abbreviations have been used,
GMS - General Medical Services
PCO - Primary Care Organisation

A

access **34, 48, 107, 110, 129–139**
  advanced access *see* Advanced access
  definition 129
  finances 117, 129–130
  models, characteristics of 131t
  monitoring 138
  myths 137t
  open 131t, 134–135
  patient communication, and 137
  quality payments, and 76, 107
  targets 130–139
  troubleshooting 138–139
accountancy,
  areas of expertise 16
  profitability, and 14–17
achievement payments **78–79**
acupuncture 36
additional services **32–33, 105–106**
  opt-out prices/global sum 33t
  quality payments, and 76, 105–106
adolescent health clinics **34, 112**
advanced access **130–139**
  alternatives to 137–139
  outcomes 131t
advertising 46
affective psychoses, Read codes 98
AISMA (Association of Independent Specialist Medical
     Accountants) 17, 125
alcohol misuse services **34, 111, 115, 118–119**
annual review **81–82**
antenatal care 32
anti-coagulant monitoring **34, 111, 119**
aspiration payments 77
aspirin prophylaxis, Read codes 84
Association of Independent Specialist Medical
     Accountants (AISMA) 17, 125
asthma care,
  quality payments, and 75, 99–101
  Read codes 99, 100
asylum seekers 49
audit 13, 143
  medical audit advisory group work 36
authorship 36

B

'backlog' **130, 134**
benefits agency work 22, 36
beta-blockers, Read codes 85
bidding, out-of-hours care **71–72**
blood pressure monitoring, Read codes 83
blood tests 23
business planning 7
  meetings
    aims and objectives 18–19
    problems 19–20
  profitability, and 17–21
business structure, profitability **7–10**

C

cancer,
  quality payments, and 75, 97–98
  Read codes 97
canvassing 46
capacity **132**
  hidden 133
  matching demand 134–135
cardiology 48
Carr–Hill allocation formula **31, 32, 47, 68**
cervical screening **32, 33t**
  quality payments, and 76, 106
child health surveillance **32, 33t**
  quality payments, and 76, 106
childhood immunisations **32, 33t**
  provision, financial value of 117
  targets 34, 110
cholesterol measurement, Read codes 84
chronic disease management 57
  quality payments *see* Quality payments
chronic obstructive pulmonary disease (COPD),
  quality payments
    and 75, 94–95
  Read codes 94, 95
claims 14
clinical data recording **11–12, 143–144**
clinical quality areas,
  practice management, and 27
  see also Quality payments
collaborative work **46–48**
committee fees 36
communication *see* Patient communication
community in-patient care 116
community psychiatric care 112
computerisation *see* Information technology
consultations, quality payments 76
contingency plans **135–136**
contraception services 23
contraceptive services **32, 33t**
  quality payments, and 76, 106
contracting (services) out 33
contracts *see* General Medical Services (GMS) practice,
    new contract; General Medical Services (GMS)
    practice, old contract
co-operatives, out-of-hours care **48, 65, 72–73**
coronary heart disease, secondary prevention **75, 82–85**
cosmetic surgery 40
cottage hospitals, cover for **34, 112**
customised searches 13
customised templates *see* Information technology

D

data recording **11–12, 143–144**
delegation **23, 42**
demand, matching capacity **134–135**
demand profiling 132
depression services **34, 111**
  provision, financial value of 119
depressive disorders, Read codes 98
dermatology services 49
diabetes care **48, 62**
  quality payments, and 75, 81, 90–94

directed enhanced services 34, 110–111
  provision, financial value of 117–118, 130
directorships 36
disciplinary review panel 36
dispensing 27
district nursing services 71
diversity 22–26, 31–50
  advantages 22, 35
  GMS, range of services 31–35
    additional 32–33
    enhanced 33–35, 109–121
    essential 31–32
  GP specialists 48–49
  opportunities, relating to 22–23
  pitfalls 43
  practices (other), working with 46–48
  principles of 42
  private work *see* Private work
doctors, salaried *see* Salaried doctors
drug company collaborations 22, 36
drug misuse services 34, 111, 115
  provision, financial value of 119–120

E

ear, nose and throat (ENT) services 49
echocardiograms, Read codes 86
education *see* Staff training
elderly care 48
electronic claims 14
EMIS 11, 143
endoscopy services 49
enhanced services 33–35, 61, 109–121
  directed *see* Directed enhanced services
  diversity, and 115–116
  financial analysis, and 109–110
  local 34–35, 112–113
  national *see* National enhanced services
  profit, calculated *vs.* actual 114–115
  types 110–114
  value of 117–121
epilepsy care,
  quality payments, and 75, 96
  Read codes 96
essential services 31–32
examinations service 37
exclusions (exception reporting), quality payments 79
exercise testing, Read codes 83
expertise, buying in 46
expert witness work 36

F

family planning services 23
fees calculation, private patients 41
financial planning 27
  business plans 7
  see also Accountancy; Income generation; Profitability
    (ideal practice)
first response care 34, 112
  provision, financial value of 120
flu vaccination *see* Influenza immunisations

G

General Medical Services (GMS) practice,
  new contract
    accounts, and *see* Accountancy
    collaborative work 46–48

financial potential of 3
general practice, future under 57
general practice income, factors affecting 61
history of 2–3
ideal structure, factors dictating 8, 9
negotiation of 2
Personal Medical Services, switching from 127–128
services, range of *see* Diversity
old contract
  inadequacies of 2
  income under 1, 3
General Practice Assessment Questionnaire (GPAQ) 105,
  159–163
G-grade nurses 56
ghost patients, quality payments 80, 82
global sum payment 31, 32, 61
GMS baseline 123
growth funding 124

H

health care assistants 56
holistic care, quality payments 81, 106
home cover, nursing 112
homeless people, enhanced care of 34, 49, 112, 116
  provision, financial value of 120
hospice work 36
hospitals, cottage 34, 112
hospital work 36
hypertension,
  quality payments, and 75, 89–90
  Read codes 89
hypothyroidism,
  quality payments, and 75, 96–97
  Read codes 97

I

immediate care 34, 112
  provision, financial value of 120
immunisations 32, 33t
  influenza *see* Influenza immunisations
  see also Childhood immunisations
Improving Practice Questionnaire (IPQ) 105, 164–166
income generation 1–2, 26–28
  cost comparison 69
  maximising NHS fees 22–23
  potential 28–29
  private work *see* Private work
  remuneration, and 25
  sources 9, 24–25
independent tribunal service 36
influenza immunisations 34, 110
  income/costs 113–114, 115, 117
  Read codes 85
information technology 16
  audit 13
  clinical data recording 11–12, 143–144
  computer resources 12, 143–144
    quality data recording 78, 79
  electronic claims 14
  profitability, and 10–14
  quality payments, and 10, 78
  searches, customised 13
  templates, customised 11–12, 12, 79
    medico-legal reports 38
injuries, minor *see* Minor injury services
in-patient care 116

InPractice Systems   143, 144
intra-partum care   34, 111, 116
   provision, financial value of   120
intrauterine contraceptive device (IUCD) fitting   34, 111, 116
   provision, financial value of   119
ischaemic heart disease, secondary prevention   75, 82–85

L
lateral thinking   20
leadership   52
leaflets   121
left ventricular dysfunction, quality payments   75, 85–86
litigation   42
local enhanced services   34–35, 112–113
loyalty payments   141–142

M
management consultancy   17–19
maternity services   32, 33t, 34
   quality payments, and   76, 106
medical accountancy see Accountancy
medical audit advisory group work   36
medical research ethics committees   36
medicals   7, 37
medical writing   23
medicines management, quality payments   76, 104
medico-legal reports   22, 24, 38–40
   sample   145–149
mental health   49
   quality payments, and   75, 98–99
   Read codes   98, 99
mergers   46, 56
micro-albuminuria testing, Read codes   92
Minimum Practice Income Guarantee (MPIG)   31, 61
minor injury services   34, 71, 112
   provision, financial value of   120–121
minor surgery   2, 32, 33t
   advanced   34, 116
   provision, financial value of   118
multiple pathology, quality payments   80–81
multiple sclerosis services   34, 111
   provision, financial value of   121
musculoskeletal care   49
myocardial infarction, Read codes   85

N
national enhanced services   34, 111–112
   provision, financial value of   118–121
National Primary Care Development Team   130
near-patient testing   34, 112
   provision, financial value of   121
neurological screening, Read codes   92
new contract see General Medical Services (GMS)
      practice, new contract
NHS Direct/NHS24   70
NHS Executive website   125
NHS Primary Care website   125
nurse practitioners   56
nurses see Practice nurses
nursing home cover   112

O
occupational health services   22, 36
old contract see General Medical Services (GMS) practice,
      old contract

open access   13t1, 137–139
opting-out,
   out-of-hours care   see Out-of-hours care
   prices/global sum, additional services   33t
   provision of services   34, 112
organisational indicators, quality payments   75–76,
      101–104
out-of-hours care   7, 23, 32, 33t, 126
   bidding   71–72
   collaborative work   46
   competition   70–71
   co-operatives   48, 65, 72–73
   definition of   67
   opting-out
      financial implications of   63, 68–69
      PCO, working for   69–70
   pricing   72
   remote/rural areas   68
   salaries   73

P
palliative care   49
paramedics   71
partnerships   8, 57
   aims and priorities of   6
   merging/splitting   8, 16, 18
   practice vs.   63–64
patient communication,
   access, and   133
   quality payments, and   75, 102
patient experience indicators, quality payments   105
patient records, quality payments and   101–102
patient satisfaction questionnaires   159–166
patient surveys,
   quality payments, and   76
   satisfaction questionnaires   159–166
pensions   16, 17, 22
Personal Medical Services (PMS)   18, 123–128
   advice, sources of   125
   contract negotiation   124–125
   financial benefits of   126–127
   pilots   123
   proposals   125–126
   switching back to GMS from   127–128
pharmaceutical company collaborations   22, 36
pilots' licences provision   36
police surgeon work   36
postnatal care   32
practice   61–66
   change, opportunities for   64–65
   economy of scale   61–62
   large, downside of   63
   management, quality payments and   76, 103–104
   medical staffing numbers   62
   partnership vs.   63–64
   profitability see Profitability (ideal practice)
practice managers   57
   role of   47, 62
practice nurses   52, 55, 57
   nurse practitioners   56
   quality payments, and   77, 79
premises   26, 27
   letting   113
   planning   16
preparation payments   77
Pricare   125, 126

pricing, out-of-hours care 72
Primary Care Agencies (PCAs) 14
Primary Care collaborative 130
Primary Care Organisations (PCOs),
 approach to 112
 board/meetings 36
 board work/meetings 23
 computerisation 11
 opting out 67, 69–70
private work 28, 35–46
 blood tests 23
 fees calculation 41
 insurance medicals 7, 37
 medico-legal reports 22, 34, 38–40
  sample 145–150
 NHS work, principles of combining with 41–42
 patient expectations 40–41
 pitfalls 43
 practice income, and 35
 vasectomies see Vasectomies, private service
problem-solving 20
profitability (ideal practice) 5–29
 accountancy 14–17
 business planning 17–21
 business structure 7–10
 diversity see Diversity
 ethos 5–7
 income generation see Income generation
 information technology, and 10–14
 maximisation of 21
 potential income 28–29
 working practices 21
protected time 28, 54
psychiatric care provision 112

Q
quality information preparation 34
 provision, financial value of 117
quality payments 61, 75–108
 access 76, 107, 130
 additional services 76, 105–106
 asthma care 75, 99–101
 cancer care 75, 97–98
 cervical screening 76, 106
 child health surveillance 76, 106
 chronic disease management 75, 82–101
  annual review, establishment of 81–82
 computer templates 12, 79
 consultations, and 76
 contraceptive services, and 76, 106
 coronary heart disease, secondary prevention 75, 82–85
 diabetes care 75, 81, 90–94
 education/training 102
 epilepsy care 75, 96
 exclusions (exception reporting) 79
 ghost patients, and 80, 82
 holistic care 81, 106
 hypertension 75, 89–90
 hypothyroidism 75, 96–97
 information technology, and 10, 78
 left ventricular dysfunction 75, 85–86
 maternity services 76, 106
 maximum available 54, 76–77
 medicines management 76, 104
 mental health 75, 98–99
 methods of 77–79

multiple pathology 80–81
organisational indicators 75–76, 101–104
patient communication 75, 102
patient experience indicators 105
patient records 101–102
practice management 76, 103–104
practice nurses, and 77, 79
quality practice payment 106–107
Read codes see Read codes
significant event analysis (SEA) 103
stroke/transient ischaemic attack 75, 86–89
troubleshooting 108
see also Quality information preparation; Quality scores
quality practice payment 106–107
quality scores 62, 63
 maximum payment available 54
questionnaires 81
 patient satisfaction 159–166

R
Read codes 12
 aspirin prophylaxis 84
 asthma 99, 100
 beta-blockers 85
 blood pressure monitoring 83
 cancer 97
 cholesterol measurement 84
 COPD 94, 95
 depressive disorders 98
 diabetes 90, 92
 echocardiograms 86
 epilepsy 96
 exclusions (exception reporting) 79
 exercise testing 83
 hypertension 89
 hypothyroidism 97
 influenza immunisations 85
 mental health 98, 99
 micro-albuminuria testing 92
 myocardial infarction 85
 neurological screening 92
 schizophrenic disorders 98
 seasonal affective disorder 98
 smoking cessation 83, 100
 spirometry 95
 stroke/transient ischaemic attack 86
recruitment issues 16
Red Book 31
 basic practice allowance, rules 8
 computer systems, under 14
 seniority payments, under 141–142
 small practices, under 65
remote/rural areas, services in 34, 67, 112
 out-of-hours care 68
rents, reimbursement 26
research contracts 23
retainer 36
retirement issues 16
review panel (disciplinary) 36

S
salaried doctors, use of 7–8
 advantages 54–55, 62
 cost of 47
 disadvantages 55
salicylate prophylaxis, Read codes 84

same-day appointments 137
Saturday morning surgeries 34, 112
    contract pricing 70
schizophrenic disorders, Read codes 98
SCOT (Strengths, Challenges, Opportunities and Threats)
    analysis 10
screening,
    cervical see Cervical screening
    refusal of 79
Screening Patient Health in an Interactive Environment
    (SOPHIE) 144
searches, customised 13
seasonal affective disorder, Read codes 98
semenalysis 44
seniority payments/scales 141–142
sexual health services 34, 111
    provision, financial value of 121
significant event analysis (SEA) 103
skill mix planning 51–59
    financial perspective 52–54
    pitfalls 53–54
    practice workforce structures 54–59
    traditional models 51–52
smoking cessation 48
    Read codes 83, 100
SOPHIE (Screening Patient Health in an Interactive
    Environment) 144
specialists 48–49
spirometry 47–48
    Read codes 95
sports medicine 22, 36
staff training 13, 27, 36, 48, 116, 23
    quality payments, and 76
standards 42
Strengths, Challenges, Opportunities and Threats (SCOT)
    analysis 10
stress 7
stroke/transient ischaemic attack,
    quality payments, and 75, 86–89
    Read codes 86
Structured Data Areas 144
subletting 26

summative assessments 36
superannuation 16, 17, 22
surgery, minor see Minor surgery
surveys see Patient surveys

T
take-overs 46
tax 22
    planning 16
teaching 36
telephone consultations, shaping demand 133
templates, customised see Information technology
Torex 11, 143, 144
traditional model of care 51–52
    access 131t
transient ischaemic attack see Stroke/transient ischaemic
    attack
travel clinics 36
travel vaccination 23
triage 56, 133, 134

U
urgent appointments, advanced access 130
V
vasectomies, private service 10
    advertising 46
    cost-effectiveness 42
    costs of provision 45t
    equipment needed 44–45
    financial rewards of 43
    paperwork 151–157
    setting up 43–46
    surgical skills required 44
        training for 49
violent patient provision 34, 110, 115, 118
Vision 11, 144

W
walk-in centres 71
whiplash injury 24, 38
'wisdom and experience' payments 141–142
working practices, profitability 21

Your professional development doesn't stop when you start in practice...

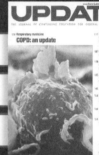

- ■ A fortnightly update on the most recent clinical developments
- ■ Practical advice and guidance on diagnosis, treatment and management
- ■ A continuing education programme designed for the busy primary care professional

Note to GPs practising in the UK: you are entitled to receive *Update* free of charge.
Please call 020 8652 8454 if you are not being sent your copy of *Update* on a regular basis.

Subscription Order Form

Title (Dr/Mr/Mrs/Miss/Ms) _____ Initial _____ Surname _____

Job title _____

Practice name _____

Address _____

_____

_____

Postcode _____ Country _____

Tel no _____ Mobile _____

Fax no _____

So that we can keep you up to date with related information, please complete the line below with your email address.
If you do not wish to receive relevant offers and information from other selected companies by email please cross here ☐

E-mail _____

Thank you for your order, please send this form and your payment to the FREEPOST address below (no stamp required in the UK). Allow up to 28 days for your first issue to arrive.

Post   *Update* Subscriptions, FREEPOST RCC2619, Haywards Heath, RH16 3BR, UK.
Telephone   +44 (0)1444 445566
Fax   +44 (0)1444 445447
Email   rbi.subscriptions@qss-uk.com

	UK Europe	Worldwide (airmail)	
1 year	£105	£128/€211	£183
2 years	£189	£230/€380	£329
3 years	£268	£326/€538	£467

(Rates valid until 31/12/03)

3 Ways to Subscribe

1   Cheque made payable to *Update* for _____

2   Please debit my Switch/Delta/Visa/Mastercard/Amex/Diners Club card
(please circle) with the amount of _____

Card no: ☐☐☐☐ ☐☐☐☐ ☐☐☐☐ ☐☐☐☐ ☐

Expiry date ☐☐ / ☐☐   Valid from ☐☐ / ☐☐   Issue no ☐

☐ Switch/Delta/applicable to certain credit cards

Signature _____ Date _____

3   Invoice me. Purchase order no. _____

If you are registered for VAT, please supply VAT reg. no. _____